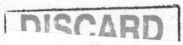

AIDS as an Apocalyptic Metaphor in North America

In a single decade, AIDS has grown to pandemic proportions. The combined forces of medical research and public education have thus far failed to halt the spread of the disease, which remains mysterious, stigmatizing, and fatal. In this highly original study, Susan Palmer explores the healing practices, metaphors, and apocalyptic fantasies of various religious, racial, and sexual minority groups as they respond to the AIDS threat.

Palmer looks at the response to AIDS by specific groups ranging from white and black identity movements and gay spirituality circles to communal and millenarian cults. Her study reveals a proliferation of AIDS metaphors that refer variously to medieval plagues, social disorder, decline of the nuclear family, and supernatural powers. She argues that the human body tends to become a symbol that mirrors the social body, and she finds this process especially dramatic in persecuted marginal groups.

Well known as a researcher and writer on new religious movements in Europe and North America, Susan Palmer brings experience and insight to this study of the metaphors surrounding alternative spirituality and sexuality.

SUSAN PALMER is a professor in the Department of Religion at Dawson College in Montreal.

AIDS

as an
Apocalyptic Metaphor in North America

SUSAN PALMER

UNIVERSITY OF TORONTO PRESS
Toronto Buffalo London

© University of Toronto Press Incorporated 1997
Toronto Buffalo London
Printed in Canada

ISBN 0-8020-0662-0 (cloth)
ISBN 0-8020-7616-5 (paper)

∞

Printed on acid-free paper

Canadian Cataloguing in Publication Data

Palmer, Susan J.
  AIDS as an apocalyptic metaphor in North America

  Includes bibliographical references.
  ISBN 0-8020-0662-0 (bound)   ISBN 0-8020-7616-5 (pbk.)

  1. AIDS (Disease) — Religious aspects. 2. AIDS (Disease) – North America.
  3. Religious minorities – North America – Attitudes.   I. Title.

  RC607.A26P34 1997   291.1'78321969792   C96-931807-3

University of Toronto Press acknowledges the financial assistance
to its publishing program of the Canada Council and the Ontario
Arts Council.

To my father, Dr Leslie Lamonte Palmer,
whose poetry, humour, and medical tales
prepared me for this work

Contents

Acknowledgments

I would like to thank the Canada Council for the Explorations grant that enabled me to pursue the idea that led to this book. I am grateful to all the people in these various religions who helped me gather and understand the material and for the encouragement I received from Tom Robbins, Fred Bird, and Charles Davis. Finally, I applaud the courage and creativity of the PWAs I met and read about.

ONE

AIDS Metaphors and Body Symbols

*Why Religious Minorities? Douglas's 'Purity' versus 'Pollution'
Theories; Nomization, Stigmatization, and Metaphorical Thinking;
Images, Associations, and Practical Solutions; Six Strategical
Responses from the Margins of Religion; Meanings and Margins*

The work that follows is not about AIDS (acquired immune deficiency sydrome), the disease. This book explores religious responses to AIDS and, as such, focuses on how people think and
feel about a new and mysterious illness. The statements appearing
in the literature of religious minorities since 1985 could hardly be
described as a series of medical bulletins. They do, however, en-
compass such vast and basic issues as love, death, sex, health, and
humanity's place in the universe. We shall see that, in the process
of trying to create meaning out of a baffling, catastrophic malady,
many of these alternative spiritual traditions remain distrustful of
doctors and suspicious of public health authorities, preferring to
interpret AIDS as a sign (of some imminent supernatural event) or
as a metaphor (for social disorder or inferior consciousness).

The intention behind this survey, therefore, is to study the metaphors, healing practices, and apocalyptic fantasies of religious
minorities as they respond to the threat of AIDS. The theoretical
approach to this material will be an anthropological one, and the
source of inspiration for making sense out of these spiritual interpretations of a contagious disease will be found in Mary Douglas's
analysis of purity rituals and pollution fears in African tribes
(Douglas, 1966). Also central to this study is the hypothesis that
the peculiar features of AIDS appear to invite what Susan Sontag
(1978) has called 'metaphorical thinking,' and that when one examines the statements issuing from religious, racial, or sexual minority groups, the underlying concern is the need to redefine,

strengthen, or rationalize the boundaries between a small society and the larger, surrounding one.

Why Religious Minorities?

I have chosen to concentrate on the literature and revelations of religious minorities – as opposed to mainstream churches – for the following reasons. First, their statements tend to be more extreme, more overtly moralistic and poetic than those issuing from more orthodox sources. Charismatic prophets seem to feel less self-conscious while waxing metaphorical than Catholic cardinals, Anglican bishops, or Protestant ministers, all of whom often sound wishy-washy and inhibited in their public pronouncements on AIDS.

Secondly, many of these alternative religions are already sensitive to the process of social stigmatization because many of them have been labelled cults, their holy men have been caricatured or demonized by the press, their successful evangelical activity has been dismissed as brainwashing, and their members have been kidnapped and subjected to the indignities of 'deprogramming.' For this reason it is interesting to watch their reactions to a new and growing stigmatized group: people with AIDS (PWAs).

Third, these groups exhibit an intense concern for purity and boundaries: the boundaries of the human body, which they guard by observing dietary and sexual taboos, and the boundaries of their social body, which struggles to maintain its integrity in the face of external persecution and the temptation to assimilate into the larger social fabric.

Fourth, millenarians and utopians in the past have often sought to restructure radically the relations between the sexes and have fostered new patterns of family life based on religious ideals, such as new visions of the godhead or prophecies of imminent global destruction. Often their unorthodox interpretations of the Fall and the consequences of sin have led them to hope for perfect health and extraordinary longevity. We will never know what the eighteenth-century messiah, Ann Lee, or the nineteenth-century prophet, Joseph Smith, might have said about AIDS, but the same preoccupation with locating the mystical link between sexual and spiritual desire appears to be shaping the budding cultures of contemporary utopians. The statements on AIDS issuing from these new communal and millenarian movements, therefore, can be understood only within the framework of their eschatologies and patterns of sexuality. The hidden spiritual relationships among sex, death, and health – themes that fascinated nineteenth-century prophets – are explored in the myths and metaphors of modern prophets when they talk about AIDS. These metaphors are interesting from a sociological standpoint, because often they are sensitive indicators of how these spiritual communities see themselves in relation to the larger society.

This study also includes the spiritual responses of sexual minorities (gays) and racial minorities (African-Americans and White Supremacists). The expanding margins between what is considered normal or fully human, and what is feared as 'other' in the popular, secular sphere of our culture are explored in two forms of popular culture: science fiction and horror cinema, and media portraits of the virus and its victims.

In order to demonstrate how AIDS metaphors are used as a boundary-maintenance strategy, my approach will be as follows:

1. The relevance of Mary Douglas's theories to understanding the 'pollution fears' evoked by AIDS-contaminated bodily fluids will be explained.

2. Insights into why AIDS is often treated as a metaphor might be gleaned from the thoughts of Peter Berger, Peter Conrad, and Susan Sontag on nomization, stigmatization, and illness.

3. The *images* and *associations* with AIDS found in new religious literature will be discussed, and the various shapes of the religious groups featured in this study, particularly in terms of their relationship with their host society, will be described.

4. Six strategical responses to the AIDS threat found among the

groups featured in this study will be outlined and will form
the basis for organizing the material in the ensuing chapters.

Douglas's 'Purity' versus 'Pollution' Theories

Douglas's well-known anthropological work, *Purity and Danger*,
was published in 1966, but her insights into body rituals and ideas
of contagion bear an almost uncanny relevance to the attitudes
towards AIDS documented in this book. The most interesting
points she raises, for our purposes, are:

1.   that there is a correspondence between notions of hygiene and
     spiritual pollution,

2.   that ideas about dirt, purity, and contagion mirror the structure
     and hierarchy of the larger social system,

3.   that the human body, with its entrances and exits, is often a
     source of symbols for the threatened boundaries of a society.

Douglas seeks to demonstrate, through an analysis of cross-
cultural concepts of dirt and pollution, that the line between sanctity and sanitation tends to be fuzzy in any society, whether tech-
nologically advanced or stone-age. She also argues that concepts
of pollution and dirt, while differing in substance between primitives and ourselves, do not necessarily differ in function, for any
social organization is based on lines that divide individuals, classes, and groups from each other. Douglas challenges the notion
that there is a clear distinction between *our* killing germs and *their*
(the 'primitives') warding off evil spirits. 'Dirt' she defines at the
outset of her book simply as 'matter out of place.' She questions
some of the condescending attitudes of the early anthropologists
such as Sir James Frazer and Robertson Smith towards primitive
societies, particularly their distinctions among magic, science, and
religion. Her advice to them is: 'we shall not attempt to expect to
understand other people's ideas of contagion, sacred or secular,
until we have confronted our own.'

This maxim would apply to our investigation of religious responses to AIDS, and the tendency observed in the secular public to dismiss religious leaders' statements on AIDS as irrational while assuming that the attitudes of doctors and journalists towards PWAs are any less fearful, hysterical, or superstitious.

Douglas's second book, *Natural Symbols* (1973), presents the notion that the human body is often treated as a 'natural symbol' of the social body, and that the body's orifices, which are carefully guarded or purified by means of purity rituals, often mirror the exits and entrances of the social body. When the social body is threatened from without, Douglas argues, the sense of threat to the social order is frequently reflected in its members' obsessive concern with bodily purity.

It appears to be a universal phenomenon that body orifices and the viscous fluids that issue from them are 'thought to be invested with power and danger' (Douglas, 1966:121). Thus, it is not only primitives and modern religious people (viewed by some as 'neo-primitives') who fear bodily fluids. Since the advent of AIDS, this phenomenon has been observed to be operating in the medical world, the police force, and the public schools. Media stories that bear witness to modern, secular varieties of pollution fears also underline their irrational element. The reactions to PWAs, for example, do not necessarily conform to what are generally understood to be the scientific facts concerning the transmission of the human immunodeficiency virus (HIV). In a similar vein, the responses of different religious groups to the epidemic are equally inconsistent, for they focus on completely different body fluids as dangerous, and tend to see the source of threat looming on different horizons.

Douglas has noted the same phenomenon in her study of purity rituals and finds that tears, for example, might be considered extremely polluting in one part of India, but are deemed pure and harmless in other parts. Excrement might be used by sorcerers as a ritual instrument of harm in one tribe, whereas a neighbouring tribe would joke about it. She attempts to account for this wide variation in attitudes to body orifices and their fluids by postulating that the human body is a symbol of society and that different cultures draw on body symbolism (which is part of the common stock of symbols) selectively, so that different rituals emphasize different body parts or orifices. As an anthropologist, she considers psychological explanations of body rituals as a mere regression to infantile fantasies of control to be inadequate, because the psycho-analytical approach does not, after all, account for cultural differences. Douglas presents her 'body as symbol' thesis as follows, and its relevance to understanding religious responses to AIDS does not need to be explained:

> The body is a model which can stand for any bounded system. Its boundaries can represent any boundaries which are threatened or precarious. The body is a complex structure. The functions of its different parts and their relation afford a source of symbols for other complex structures. We cannot possibly interpret rituals concerning excreta, breast milk, saliva and the rest unless we are prepared to see in the body a symbol of society, and to see the powers and dangers credited to social structure reproduced in small on the human body. (Douglas, 1966:115)

Douglas's theories, therefore, give us some insights into why AIDS is evidently such an irresistible topic for religious leaders. In the life of society, she observes, pollution ideas reinforce social pressures: '. . . certain moral values are upheld and certain social rules defined by beliefs on dangerous contagion, as when the glance or touch of an adulterer is held to bring illness to his neighbours or his children.' This passage might have been a direct comment on the pronouncements of evangelists Billy Graham, Jimmy Swaggart, and Moody Adams, who exploit the terror and mystery that obfuscate the AIDS crisis in order to uphold traditional Protestant and American middle-class standards of sexual behaviour. The passage below might have been addressed to these leaders and to all those who adhere to the 'wrath of God' thesis:

> the ideal order of society is guarded by dangers which threaten transgressors. These danger-beliefs are as much threats which one man uses to coerce another as dangers which he himself fears to

incur by his own lapses from righteousness. They are a strong language of mutual exhortation. At this level the laws of nature are dragged in to sanction the moral code: this kind of disease is caused by adultery, that by incest; this meteorological disaster is the effect of political disloyalty, that the effect of impiety. The whole universe is harnessed to men's attempts to force one another into good citizenship. (Douglas, 1966:3)

Nomization, Stigmatization, and Metaphorical Thinking

In order to understand how and why the disease AIDS is treated as a metaphor by religious minorities, it is useful to turn to Peter Berger's thoughts on nomization. He suggests that 'the most important function of society is nomization' which creates a 'shield against terror.' Every *nomos* is 'an edifice erected in the face of the potent and alien forces of chaos' (Berger, 1969:23). Thus the social order provides a shelter from marginal situations that reveal the 'innate precariousness of all social worlds.' Death is the marginal situation *par excellence,* not only because of its obvious threat to the continuity of human relationships, but because it threatens the basic assumptions of order on which society rests. Sexual deviance is another area that provokes anomic terror. Berger notes that the sexual program of a society is taken for granted, not simply as a utilitarian or morally correct arrangement, but as an inevitable expression of human nature. He cites the 'homosexual panic' as an illustration of the terror unleashed by the denial of the program (Berger, 1969:24).

Religion, according to Berger, is 'the human enterprise by which a sacred cosmos is established' and it plays a strategic part in world construction. Since the antonym to the sacred is the profane, to be in a 'right' relationship with the sacred cosmos is to be 'protected against the nightmare threats of chaos and anomie' (Berger, 1969:26). Nomic constructions, designed to keep terror at bay, achieve their ultimate culmination – 'literally their apotheosis' (Berger, 1969:27) – in the sacred cosmos. Therefore, since each religion projects its version of the human order – including its sexual program – into the totality of being, it is understandable that a fatal, sexually transmitted disease, which is contracted through what each church defines as sexually deviant behaviour, should become a symbol of the profane.

Disease is another marginal situation to which society must respond, and Peter Conrad regards the American public's 'overblown ... irrational and pointless reaction to AIDS' (Conrad, 1986:51) as an example of the anomic terror of the profane. Conrad asserts that 'illness,' unlike 'disease' (which is a biophysical phenomenon), involves the world of subjective interpretation and meaning: 'how a culture defines an illness and how individuals experience their disorder' (Conrad, 1986:51). Therefore, he attributes the public's hysterical response to AIDS to the particular *social* features of the disease that combine to form a cultural image of AIDS that is socially devastating: 'AIDS is a disease with a triple stigma: it is connected to stigmatized groups, it is sexually transmitted, and it is a terminal disease' (Conrad, 1986:54). Conrad touches briefly on the moral and religious meaning of AIDS, and he points out that it belongs to that group of illnesses that reflect moral shame on the individuals who had the ill luck to contract them: 'Venereal diseases ... became a symbol for social disorder and moral decay – a metaphor of evil' (Conrad, 1986:56).

Susan Sontag (1978) has explored the social meaning of illness in the nineteenth century's romantic obsession with tuberculosis and in the contemporary mystique surrounding cancer. She argues that metaphorical thinking about disease tends to place the burden of guilt on the patient, and attributes this to our cowardly inclination to reduce ineluctable realities like fatal illnesses to mere psychological phenomena. *Illness as Metaphor* was published in 1978, before the identification of the AIDS virus in America, but Sontag's ideas contribute towards an understanding of popular attitudes to AIDS, particularly her observation on why certain diseases invite 'metaphorical thinking':

Any important disease whose causality is murky, and for which treatment is ineffectual, tends to be awash in significance. First, the subjects of deepest dread (corruption, decay, pollution, anomy, weakness) are identified with the disease. The disease itself becomes a metaphor. (Sontag, 1978:57)

In Sontag's more recent book, *AIDS and Its Metaphors* (1989), she continues to deplore metaphorical language that distorts the reality of AIDS and she condemns the term 'the new plague' for its implication that the virus is a deserved punishment.

If one examines the literature on AIDS issuing from contemporary spiritual movements in the light of the theories of Berger, Conrad, and Sontag, it appears inevitable that when faced with a catastrophic event involving the issues of fatal illness, sexual morality, and the outcast status of PWAs, each religious community *must* respond in an effort to bolster its own particular world construction and to reduce terror among its congregation. Since we live in a secular age in which 'reality' is multifaceted, it is also inevitable that different congregations should come up with different interpretations of the same set of events.

Images, Associations, and Practical Solutions

An examination of the body of material generated by religious, racial, and sexual minorities reveals that they have created their own images, associations, and solutions as ways of understanding that vague and threatening phenomenon known as AIDS. These images and associations operate as *condensed symbols* that refer to a much wider variety of experiences in these groups, and often convey powerful images of other realms of life. Ray Fitzpatrick (1984: 15–25), in writing of lay concepts of illness, identifies four dominant themes or metaphors that permeate folk beliefs about illness, and these vary in emphasis as one moves from culture to culture. They propose a logic of (1) degeneration, (2) blockage, (3) balance, and (4) invasion. A characteristically Western mode of interpreting illness is 'stress' – a combination of (1) and (2). All four of these lay notions of illness are found in the religiously based images of AIDS that follow.

The Central Image of AIDS

Each group has its own image of AIDS that implies the hidden moral or the supernatural origin of the disease. Some groups call it a 'plague,' others insist it is a 'punishment' for flouting the will of God or Nature. Premillennialists interpret it as a 'Sign of the Last Days' or fit it into the 'Seven Years of Tribulation' or call it the 'Armageddon in our arteries.' Natural imagery is another approach: a 'slow earthquake,' the 'tail of a comet,' or the 'birthpangs of the planet.'

The Set of Associations/Assumptions about AIDS

Many groups automatically associate AIDS with sexual promiscuity. Others insist that the important issue is not sexual behaviour but rather hygiene: that we should listen to scientists' advice on killing, sterilizing, and blocking a lethal virus. They peer through the microscope instead of wagging the finger at singles' clubs. Some church leaders ignore heterosexual philandering but focus on the more esoteric mating habits of homosexuals. Illicit drugs and shared needles might be the main concern, or blood transfusions. A few groups associate the virus primarily with racial tensions; they claim the virus was initially generated by interracial dating or that it was deliberately introduced into black ghettos with genocidal intent by white scientists. Others read it as a new chapter in an ongoing, ancient conspiracy involving Masonic lodges and Lost Atlanteans. A few fringe groups associate the virus with bestiality: zookeepers mating with dolphins, Africans with green monkeys, or extraterrestrials with *Homo sapiens*.

Solutions and Practical Strategies

What solutions are recommended? What should be done about the epidemic? Communal and utopian groups tend to advocate compulsory AIDS tests for their members and aspire to provide a paradigm of a pure and healthy community which the larger society will eventually adopt. 'Cults' and sects[1] often point out that their code of sexual ethics (whether it be celibacy, chaperoned courting, arranged marriages, or hygienic 'free love') has already solved the problem – at least for their members. Christian-based sects and small churches in their third or fourth generation tend to worry about the boundaries of the family unit and what is appropriate in sex education for teenagers. Some religious organizations are concerned about helping those afflicted with AIDS and are opening up hospices and setting up counselling services and support groups. New Age groups have formed healing circles and developed techniques of visualization and meditation for combating the progress of the virus within the sick person's body. Premillennialists tend to await supernatural intervention: the Great Physician Himself will come again to end all sin, suffering, and death. Certain UFO cults expect starships to descend in the year 2000 bearing the antidote.

Six Strategical Responses from the Margins of Religion

These various images and associations offering keys for interpreting the AIDS threat appear to fall into six distinct categories: the judgmental, the compassionate, the healing, the isolating, the threatened, and the pragmatic response. The chapters that follow analyse the characteristics of different types of religious bodies that have adopted one or more of the following responses. How these six religious responses serve to transcend death and protect the boundaries of human and social bodies from a mysterious, stigmatized 'plague' will be discussed at greater length in the ensuing chapters.

The Judgmental Response

This response is most often found among fundamentalist groups, who tend to view the disease as a form of divine punishment, as Nature's 'backlash,' as Satan's last-ditch struggle to preserve his dominion over God's Country, or as an invasion of demons (disguised as stricken homosexuals) marching up from the bowels of Hell. There is no pity or aid extended to PWAs, who are considered responsible for their fate, and consequently should be shunned. Since many of the Christian fundamentalist churches that adopt this attitude anticipate the imminent return of Christ, who will 'rapture' them to safety while the rest of the world is destroyed, they do not bother to read the latest medical reports, are apathetic concerning the prospect of finding a cure, and ignore public health authorities' statements, since they are completely confident that sticking to their moral code will protect them from contagion.

The 'Nature's backlash' interpretation of AIDS has been most eloquently voiced by the leaders of Earth First!, the radical underground environmental movement documented by Martha Lee (1995). Lee traces the development of the group's apocalyptic doctrines and gradual alienation from society, which led to the illegal activist measures of arson, bombing, tree spiking, and 'monkey-wrenching' of road equipment – and to a major FBI investigation. Christopher Manes, writing under the pseudonym, 'Miss An Thropy,' argued in the group's newsletter that the spread of AIDS was actually a fortuitous coincidence and a viable solution to the world overpopulation crisis (Manes, 1987:17). Another leader, Daniel Conner, went one step further in proposing that AIDS was Gaia's wholesome and self-protective response to the unbearable pressures of overpopulation, pollution, and species extinction. As a champion of biocentrism (the belief that the earth, as a single, living organism, needs the full complement of all her species) and of bioequality (the belief that all species are equal), he predicted that AIDS would spread among heterosexuals, that it would mutate into many strains, and that even if a cure were found, Gaia would – of necessity – create another, more virulent disease (Conner, 1987:14–16).

The Compassionate Response

The compassionate or 'Good Samaritan' response to PWAs is found in those religions that are committed in their belief structure to alleviating human suffering and may already have a well-established role as helpers of the needy and outcasts of society. Churches that can afford to be compassionate tend to be on good terms with the larger society, are institutionalized rather than charismatic in their authority patterns, and have clearly established their social boundaries. Other groups, particularly those within the gay movement, identify with PWAs, and therein lies their impulse towards compassion.

This response is characterized by a pragmatic, non-judgmental attitude towards PWAs, and by practical assistance in the form of volunteer counselling, care, and the setting up of hospices or wards. The emphasis is on group support and preparations for death rather than on attempts at faith healing. Some spiritual organizations inclined towards compassion provide meditation instruction or prayer circles to facilitate a calm acceptance of death in the midst of community support. Classes might be offered to enable PWAs to explore traditional teachings on suffering and post-death experiences, or listen to sacred narratives of the afterlife, which will help create a context of meaning or transcendence in imagining their own death. This approach includes PWAs in a community of believers.

Congregations that adopt the compassionate response do not appear overly worried about contagion. They tend to feel confident that if they observe medically approved hygienic measures and the moral guidelines of their church, they will be far removed from the threat of AIDS. These groups are often well informed concerning the latest developments in AIDS research; they take doctors' recommendations very seriously, express a faith in science, and are optimistic that it will discover a cure.

The Healing Response

This response is characterized by the notion that the right attitude or the right techniques can enable PWAs to heal themselves. The body-mind connection is stressed, magical techniques are marketed or shared, and the state of consciousness of the sick person is considered more significant than clinical data. Healing groups tend to exhibit a positive attitude towards non-procreative sexual relationships, and are consequently non-judgmental in their treatment of PWAs.

This type of response is found among churches already committed to a form of spiritual healing, such as Christian Science and the United Church of Religious Science and other descendants of the New Thought movement. It is also found in urban shamanism, in small, charismatic groups issuing from the New Age movement or the gay community. The growing market of afflicted gay successful professionals with healthy incomes, but no children to provide for, has attracted spiritual practitioners and urban shamans to set up shop. Occult remedies and esoteric rituals for PWAs are advertised. New Age therapists, channellers, and healing practitioners claim their techniques enable AIDS-stricken clients to achieve 'a relatively stable condition.' Various diet plans marketed in New Age magazines and gay newsletters that promise to bolster the immune system and – in some instances – to cure PWAs completely. New euphemisms for AIDS, such as 'life-challenging illnesses,' appear on posters. Healing circles for PWAs are advertised in occult bookshops, natural foods restaurants, and gay community centres, and which offer a synthesis of techniques that might include crystals, channelling, past life regressions, visualizations, and so on. Many of these practitioners deliberately cater to the gay community, and their literature and posters exhibit positive attitudes towards homosexuality.

The Isolating Response

Policies to exclude and isolate PWAs are found in religions that might be described as communal utopias (Kanter, 1972) or millenarian sects. These 'world rejecting' (Wallis, 1984) religions tend to be uncompromising in their policies to exclude HIV-positive people from their communities. In many of these groups, the isolating response to AIDS is a product of their apocalyptic expectations. Since they believe the Second Coming will free humankind from the consequences of original sin in the approaching millennium, AIDS is often interpreted as an external sign of those who are not of the 'elect' or who will not be 'raptured' to enjoy a relative immortality in the twenty-first century. The isolating response in its most extreme form can be found in new charismatic religions that feel their boundaries are threatened by external persecution. If they have been investigated by secular authorities, if their leader has been arrested, or if their family and economic patterns have been disrupted by legal procedures or maligned and ridiculed in the press, they are likely to intensify their concern for maintaining order and for protecting the purity and health of their members.

Those new religious movements that demand HIV tests from members or visitors are all communal in their social organization. These include the Unification Church, the Rajneesh (Osho) movement, the Northeast Kingdom Community, and The Family. These communes have evolved radically alternative gender roles and elaborate philosophies of sexuality. They have clear-cut ideas on purity and rigorously observe sexual and dietary taboos that pre-date the advent of AIDS, but that are often strangely congruent with current scientifically approved prophylactic measures. They tend to regard the virus as extremely contagious, and recommend that their members err on the side of caution – particularly in dealing with outsiders, who are perceived as careless, unaware, and potential carriers.

The Threatened Response

Groups that have fabricated conspiracy theories to explain social problems or political events, and who adhere to a self-image as a people who are superior, more fully human, the 'elect,' is God's chosen people who have a special role in history – these groups exhibit the threatened response to AIDS. Many of these conspiracy theories involve anti-Semitic sentiments and idiosyncratic forms of racism.

This response is characterized by a tendency to magnify the danger (e.g., calling it a 'pandemic' or a 'holocaust'), to combine a sophisticated grasp of the latest medical information on the virus with a strong mistrust for public health authorities, and to account for the origin and dissemination of AIDS as an age-old plot or an international conspiracy. Consequently, PWAs are not blamed; rather, they are pitied as the unwitting victims of ruthless politicians and scientists. Media reports and orthodox scientific theories are discounted or viewed with suspicion, for the solution to the AIDS threat for these groups lies in unmasking the conspiracy. Many of these groups seek to increase their political influence and to restore America to what they nostalgically perceive as its constitutional purity and justice. AIDS is therefore often a symbol for the erosian of pioneer values and the fading of the American dream.

The Pragmatic Response

The pragmatic response characterizes many religious minorities that appear to have little or nothing to say about AIDS. They exhibit no signs of metaphorical thinking and have not responded to the issue in their publications. It could be argued that religions that correspond to Wallis's 'world affirming' type (1984) are inclined to demonstrate tolerant attitudes towards homosexuals and PWAs, and prefer to leave the problem of avoiding contagion up to the individual's discretion. For these groups, AIDS is not a religiously significant issue, and their down-to-earth approach avoids moralizing.

Meanings and Margins

The morals and meanings extracted from AIDS often reflect the deepest concerns of a particular religion. The Jehovah's Witnesses point out that AIDS proves that blood transfusions are against the law of Jehovah. Arcane societies that place the consumption of body fluids – as symbols of immortality – central to their ritual life manifest an intense concern about AIDS. Vampire circles have modified their communion so that members drink their own blood from their personal cup. Gnostic groups that seek to imbibe pure spiritual knowledge through the ritual of sperm-drinking find the notion of a contaminated *gnosis* deeply threatening. The peculiar features of the virus are described such that they reinforce the sexual ethics or millenarian expectations of certain communities. Underlying these concerns, however, is the imperative to redefine social boundaries and strengthen human bonds. While congregants' statements tend to be consistent with the religious body's belief system, they often reveal as much about the social organization of the group as they do about its world view. Some groups, for example, respond to the AIDS threat by exhorting their members to protect the boundaries of the family unit. Readers of *The Plain Truth*, a publication of the Worldwide Church of God, are encouraged to reinforce the fortress of monogamy from within, whereas Plymouth Brethren and Mormons try to protect their teenagers from the amoral ambiguity and mixed messages of sex education programs in the public schools.

The most extreme 'spiritual solutions' to the 'new plague' are found in the type of religious organization that demands total commitment from its members and is the most alienated from American culture. This is the world-rejecting spiritual commune that often rejects the biological family in favour of the 'spiritual family.' It is perhaps not coincidental that all the communal groups included in this study insist on HIV tests for members and aspiring initiates. This practice might be explained as arising from a natural concern over the sharing of food and bathroom facilities, which characterizes communal life, but it could also be interpreted in sociological terms as reflecting the feelings of vulnerability or threat – what Mary Douglas calls the 'pollution fears' – of a small, persecuted religious minority.

At the other end of the spectrum (in terms of their social organization) are the quasi-religious cults, the therapeutically oriented groups or 'magic' weekend-intensive workshops that offer courses to a transient procession of clients. These 'Apprentice' groups, as Bird (1978) calls them, impart techniques that enable the adept to tap sources of power within the self or in nature that can be used for material, secular ends. Such groups locate the sacred as residing within each individual, and, in responding to AIDS, their leaders and practitioners tend to recommend medically approved prophylactic measures (e.g., condoms) to preserve their clients' physical and psychic autonomy. Often, however, they prefer to leave the problem of contagion up to the individual's discretion. The boundaries separating Apprentice groups from the larger society are porous and flimsy, since they encourage their members to be world affirming and success seeking in their orientation towards the secular world.

Each chapter that follows describes a different type of group and its unique characteristics that condition its response to AIDS. The boundaries separating these communities from the outside world vary considerably in their relative density, porousness, and flexibility.

Chapter 2 examines the thoughts on AIDS of televangelists and the leaders of small Christian churches or sects whose following are often indistinguishable from America's 'moral majority.' Whereas Jehovah's Witnesses and Mormons maintain firm boundaries between their congregation of 'co-rulers with Jehovah' or 'Saints' and the population (with lower moral standards) without, these churches have gained social credibility and are no longer branded as cults, except by fundamentalist authors of anti-heresy propaganda.

Chapter 3 explores the policies on AIDS that have evolved within communal movements: the Unification Church, the Messianic Communities, the Rajneesh, Krishna Consciousness, and others. All these spiritual communities have strict standards of sexual and dietary purity that are consistent with their communal patterns or millenarian expectations. All have suffered some degree of persecution at the hands of secular authorities or bad press from journalists.

Chapter 4 features non-communal new religious movements of the world-affirming type that offer meditation or therapeutic techniques promising members better adjustment to secular life.

Chapter 5 looks at AIDS through the eyes of those racialist religions espousing conspiracy theories.

Chapter 6 explores spiritual strategies for coping with the 'new plague' in various gay groups, and how AIDS metaphors are used to define the margins between their stigmatized community and the heterosexual culture surrounding it.

Chapter 7 argues that many of the apocalyptic fantasies and primordial fears expressed overtly in the literature of religious minorities can also be detected in popular culture: in various forms of 'secular armageddonism,' in magazine portraits of PWAs, and in cinematic sagas of sexy xenomorphs bringing extraterrestrial plagues to our planet.

Chapter 8 surveys apocalyptic themes and AIDS metaphors in the media and proposes that the American obsession with AIDS stems from a deep concern over the widening chinks in the armour of what Aries (1981) and Chidester (1990) call the 'American way of death.'

This survey will show that metaphorical thinking about AIDS often expresses the anxiety evoked by threatened boundaries. More than any other disease, AIDS crosses categories, is identified with marginal groups, and lurks in liminal places. Initially the virus defied classification, for like Augustine's definition of evil as a 'privation of good,' it manifested itself in the immune system not as a presence, but rather as an absence; a privation of the body's defences against germs. Its victims, weakened by the relentless onslaught of opportunistic diseases, appeared to die of Disease itself. People who have contracted the virus are also difficult to place within a grid of meaning. Because of the long incubation period, PWAs might be unwitting carriers who are young, beautiful, and sexually active, or they might be bedridden, emaciated, coughing patients whom no one wants to touch. In 1986, it was homosexuals, Haitians, and heroin addicts who got AIDS. By 1991 it could be anyone.

As the epidemic expands exponentially, the boundaries between 'us' (the safe and healthy) and 'them' (the sick or risky) have formed new contours. The name for these people has been changed periodically in order to remove the stigma. 'AIDS victims' sounded pathetic, 'AIDS carriers' threatening, whereas the recent 'PWA' (person with AIDS) conveys a neutral stance. As Ted Hughes (*Time*, 3 February 1992:46) points out, 'Americans want to create a sort of "linguistic Lourdes" where evil and misfortune are dispelled in the waters of euphemism.' AIDS talk is often about erecting new barriers between the sexes or restoring the crumbling edifices of meaning in our culture. Hopefully, what those lost boundaries and decaying edifices are will become clearer by the end of this study.

TWO

Christian Compassion or Condemnation?

The Worldwide Church of God, Evangelist Moody Adams, Billy Graham, Jimmy Swaggart Ministries, The Church of Jesus Christ, Scientist, The Church of the Latter-Day Saints, The Jehovah's Witnesses, The Seventh-Day Adventists, AIDS and Christian Apocalypticism

This chapter examines Christian responses to the 'new plague,' which range from the judgmental to the compassionate. The leaders of these religious movements speak from two positions: from the centre and from the margins. Preaching from the centre, tele-vangelists such as Billy Graham are intent on evangelizing the world, and so find it expedient to downplay particular views of biblical prophecy and specific prescriptions in the realm of morality. Hoping to extend their outreach across different denominations, they cultivate a disciplined participation in society and a non-separatist orientation.

Speaking from the margins are the leaders of the Christian sects. Their concern is to fortify the walls of their community so as to maintain the purity of their elite company of 'latter-day saints': their 144,000 co-rulers with Jehovah, or their Anglo-Israelite 'chosen' people. Their apocalyptic expectations are often specific and highly elaborate, and many of their leaders display an eager creativity in weaving the 'fearsome plague' into their premillennial images.

A survey of the more orthodox and well-established Christian churches' responses to AIDS (Melton, 1989) tends to support Robert Wuthnow's observations in *The Restructuring of American Religion* (1989). He claims: 'By the early 1980s, then, the lines separating religious conservatives from religious liberals had come to be drawn with a wide brush,' and he traces the decline of denominationalism as the boundaries that distinguished church bodies from each other faded and a widening chasm arose between the New Christian Right and the liberal Christians. He notes the phenomenon of churches' realigning their allegiances in respect to such issues as abortion, ordination of women, and homosexuality. Debates over these issues he explains as 'symbolic warfare' – a war that was about symbols and was waged with symbols (Wuthnow, 1989:207). As the statements presented below suggest, AIDS and its peculiar features has become a store of new ammunition in the symbolic warfare waged between the New Christian Right and the Christian liberals. As Wuthnow notes, by the early 1970s 'Morality became a kind of no man's land into which both sides launched forays,' and issues that highlighted the modern ambiguity of boundaries separating private morality and collective life – issues such as homosexuality, abortion, and AIDS – were used as weapons in the struggle to redefine cultural categories.

The sermons on AIDS cited in the first half of this chapter issue from the mouths of radio and television personalities whose job is to run revival meetings and to move their audiences to be 'born again in Christ Jesus.' Although most of them are affiliated with Baptist or Pentacostal churches, they do not have to fulfil pastoral roles nor function as administrators within the body of a church. Their warnings on AIDS, therefore, reflect their role as charismatic preachers, for their main concern is not to protect congregations but rather to move young Christians to accept Jesus into their hearts and to refrain from sinful sexual activity. Evangelists, in responding to AIDS, have been quick to point out the apparent congruity between biblical injunctions against fornication and homosexuality and the fatal consequences that have resulted from these activities since 1982. The central image often used to evoke the terror of AIDS is that of divine punishment for sexual behaviour that is against the will of God and hence is profane. Billy Graham merely hints at this and avoids finger wagging, but Moody Adams and the Worldwide Church of God are explicit on this point. Also expressed is the notion of Satan's influence – that humankind's susceptibility to sin and its corollary, AIDS, dates back to the Fall of Adam and Eve. AIDS, as a sign of the Last Days, is the other image used by evangelists. Billy Graham hints that 'it could be a

warning of something worse to come,' but Adams calls it 'an apocalyptic Armageddon in our arteries' and concurs with the Worldwide Church of God that the epidemic is a herald of the Second
Coming.

The four small churches or sects described below were founded
in nineteenth-century North America. Two of them, the Seventh-
Day Adventists and the Jehovah's Witnesses, grew out of the Mil-
lerites' adventist movement. Many of the social problems that
Christian reformers in the nineteenth century struggled to overcome through uniting their efforts in the movements for abolition,
temperance, and women's suffrage are reflected in the doctrines
and practices of these churches today. The Seventh-Day Adventists, the Mormons, and the Christian Scientists are strongly concerned with the individual's control over health and proscribe the
use of tobacco, alcohol, and caffeine. The Jehovah's Witnesses outlaw tobacco. Christian Scientists reject medical services and medicinal drugs, preferring to rely on the healing prayers of their
practitioners. Changes in the structure of the family, and in traditional sex roles in the Victorian era, resulting from the Industrial
Revolution, the U.S. Civil War, the decline of the extended family
and the rise of the nuclear family, also affected these nascent religions, which responded in various ways. Some of them feature
female prophets and founders such as Ellen G. White and Mary
Baker Eddy. Others, like the Mormons and the Witnesses, concen-
trated on strengthening the father's spiritual authority in the home.
The Latter-Day Saints (or Mormons, as they are popularly known)
exalted the role of wife, mother, homemaker as a path to salvation
and exerted considerable social and theological pressure on husbands to be good providers and responsible heads of the family.
Therefore, we find that many of the current issues surrounding the
AIDS threat – the individual's control over health, changing gender
roles, recreational drugs, and millenarian expectations – were important issues in the schismatic movements in Protestantism over
one hundred years ago.

These churches associate the AIDS virus with sexual liaisons
outside the bonds of matrimony – but also with poor hygiene.
Consequently, their solution to the AIDS problem encompasses

strict obedience to their code of sexual behaviour, but also good medical care for the afflicted and proper hygienic precautions for their caregivers.

AIDS is dramatically conceptualized in these churches as a plague 'of fearsome dimensions,' as a 'leprosy' and 'pestilence,' a 'pale horse of death and deadly plague.' Only the Christian Scientists provide no imagery or concepts whatsoever, since they consider illness to be an illusion.

The Worldwide Church of God (Church of Tomorrow)

The late Herbert W. Armstrong died before the advent of AIDS, and although he started out as a successful radio and TV evangelist, certain features of his church suggest that the Worldwide Church of God (WWCG) might have more in common with the nineteenth-century Christian sectarian churches described below than with the audiences of current televangelists.

The message preached by Armstrong was a curious blend of Christian fundamentalism and eccentric interpretation of biblical prophecy, based on the notion of British Israelism as the Master Key that unlocked the scriptures. Armstrong claimed to be the 'Only Apostle for our Time,' divinely appointed to spread the 'advance news' in the last days of the world. His apocalyptic theory was that the Second Coming would occur in January 1972, and 'while Satan visited war and pestilence on the world, God's people would take refuge in Petra, Palestine, until Jesus had given Satan his cosmic comeuppance and transformed the world into a kind of urbanized Eden' (Martin, 1982:59).

Members of the WWCG must observe the dietary laws of the Jews, are forbidden to remarry if divorced, and must separate from their spouse and move one state away if they have already remarried before joining the church. Sickness is regarded as the penalty for sin, and members cannot take medicine or see a doctor but must resort to prayer, as healing is God's forgiveness.

In the articles on AIDS appearing in WWCG's publication, *The Plain Truth*, it is clearly stated that the 'new plague' is a punishment from God:

> Do not think that God is ignorant about all this! To the contrary,
> God is going to respond . . . The Creator, for now, is letting human
> beings reap the natural consequences of their own ways of living.
> (*The Plain Truth*, November 1985:40)

AIDS is linked to the biblical prophecy:

> The apostle Paul was inspired to write that 'in the last days perilous
> times will come' . . . That includes serious diseases. (*The Plain Truth*,
> March 1988:6)

> Few realize the Bible prophesied the alarming social disease epidem-
> ics reported in this article. Note the prophecy of Deuteronomy 28:
> 'The Lord will bring upon you and your offspring extraordinary
> afflictions . . . and sickness everlasting. (*The Plain Truth*, November
> 1985:40)

The Church's standards of sexual conduct are restated as based
on divine authority:

> God's laws were designed to protect the family unit . . . disobeyed
> they bring unimaginable social curses! . . . God made the human
> body . . . the male and female sex organs . . . are not made for lust,
> perversion or promiscuity. (*The Plain Truth*, November 1985:40)

AIDS therefore is the consequence of flouting this authority:

> the virus is not new in existence. Like many other disease pathogens
> [it comes] to the fore when God's revealed spiritual and natural laws
> of proper living are violated. (*The Plain Truth*, March 1988:6)

The origins of AIDS are traced back to Adam and Eve when 'the
spirit and attitude of rebellion against God . . . had entered their
minds.' Since then, 'God has allowed humanity 6,000 years to develop various cultures under Satan's sway – and experience the
results.' AIDS is one of the results, since:

> Satan has worked in human cultures to pervert human attitudes,

emotions and relationships . . . Satan and his host work to implant in unwary human minds selfish moods, attitudes and feelings – including improper sexual feelings. . . (*The Plain Truth*, March, 1988:5)

Finally, the WWCG work the AIDS theme into their apocalyptic theory by anticipating the Second Coming as the only cure:

To stop the growing plague . . . Jesus Christ must come with the full power and authority from God the Father to put down sin and establish the government and laws of God over all nations. (*The Plain Truth*, March 1988:6)

Evangelist Moody Adams

The Louisiana evangelist, Moody Adams, adopts a dispensationist approach to the virus in his book, *AIDS: You Just Think You're Safe* (Adams, 1986). Adams emphatically states: 'This Divine revelation makes it extremely clear that God does use diseases to punish people' (Adams, 1986:151), and he quotes passages from Deuteronomy to prove his point.

The Book of Revelation holds a 'preview of a horrible epidemic preceding our Lord's return,' Adams notes, and quotes the verses on the seven angels pouring out vials of wrath upon the earth. The cancer Kaposi's sarcoma, which afflicts many PWAs, is the predicted 'festering sores' of Revelation (Adams, 1986:224). He presents the virus as a microscopic Armageddon: 'AIDS is turning into an Apocalyptic Armageddon in our arteries, as deadly and as prophetic as any battle field weapon,' and predicts that the disease will become a colossal epidemic, at which point Jesus will descend:

As terrible as the AIDS epidemic is, there is hope. The Bible's prophecies assure us that God is still on his throne and everything is proceeding according to His plan and Christ is coming soon. After the last disease, deliverance . . . After man's mess comes God's Messiah. The worst of times will usher in the best of times. Prophecy is the light at the end of AIDS's dark tunnel . . . Ancient Prophecies whisper to all followers of Christ, 'Jesus Christ is coming. Victory is on its way.' (Adams, 1986:232)

In the chapter 'The Birth of a Monster' Adams asserts that the American strain of AIDS originated from the homosexual act, and spread through 'Fourteen Sex Acts That Are Real Killers' which he proceeds to describe with gusto, such as this 'water sport':

> another variation, practiced in some bars in New York and Miami, was having urine piped down from the second floor rest rooms and sprayed over the first floor patrons. 'The homosexuals involved found this very exciting' said Bray. (Adams, 1986:91)

Much of Adams's book is devoted to denunciation of homosexuals whose 'filthy sex habits' are linked to 'the devil who causes the disease' (Adams, 1986:229).

AIDS is also linked to 'humanist teachers who do not believe in moral absolutes' and 'liberal preachers who scoff at the Bible's moral laws.' 'AIDS is just that: the liberals' leprosy.' It is 'God's curse on those who have perverted scripture.' Adams then presents the reader with a long list of individuals who have evoked God's ire, who are mainly liberal bishops in the Episcopal Church:

> God is angry with ... Reverend Sylvia Pennington, the author of *Good News for Modern Gays* ... God is angry with Bishop Moore [who said] 'AIDS is not God's vengeance on the homosexual community' ... God is furious with the Universal fellowship of Metropolitan Community Churches, a homosexual denomination. (Adams, 1986:175–6)

Billy Graham

Billy Graham, born in 1918 in North Carolina, preaches a message that stands solidly in the conservative wing of orthodox Protestant thought. Primary is the conviction that all are sinners needing salvation. Individuals who do not recognize this need are without hope for eternal life. Social ills are the products of individual sinners, and the more sin prevails, the closer we approach the Apocalypse. Hence we are living in a time of crisis, and the solution is not social reform but rather the conversion of individuals to a commitment in Christ. The extraordinary response and subsequent publicity he received during an evangelistic campaign he conducted in Los Angeles in 1949 catapulted Billy Graham into national fame (Lippy, 1989). Lippy accounts for the evangelist's popularity as follows:

> Graham's confidence that a personal decision to accept Christ as Savior resolved all problems, his cry for a fresh national commitment to morality, his conviction that the United States had a God-ordained role in human affairs, and his biting condemnation of communism struck home. His preaching made the realities of postwar life understandable and offered hope for the future. (Lippy, 1989:180)

Billy Graham's thoughts on AIDS are presented in the October 1987 edition of *Decision*, published in Winnipeg, Canada. A handsome young college couple adorn the cover; a thoughtful, worried expression darkens both their faces. Graham sets the tone with a scary anecdote:

> A guest told of a Hollywood actor who stepped out on his wife to pick up a beautiful woman in a bar. He slept with her that night, only to wake in the morning to find her gone. Scrawled in lipstick on the bathroom mirror were the words: 'Welcome to the wonderful world of AIDS!' Can you imagine how he felt?

Then he warns that the disease is a 'pandemic' and that it might even pose a greater threat to the nation than 'an ideology we are afraid of, or even nuclear war.' The possibility of the 'wrath of God' is touched on, but Graham prefers to focus on the issue of premarital and extramarital sex:

> It may be a judgment of God upon us. I can't say that for certain, because only God would know that. But something is happening to us, paying us back for our promiscuity and our free way of life, in

which God has certain rules and regulations outlined in the Scriptures. Or it could be just a warning from God of something worse yet to come.

Graham cites passages and stories from the Bible in which death or stoning are the penalties for adultery. He also criticizes the modern tendency to blame the woman and not the man, and reminds us of the sins we must confront at the Last Judgment. Asked if he 'believes in sex,' Graham replies, 'I wouldn't be here if it weren't for sex,' and comments on the profane versus the sacred use of sexuality:

Today sex is used to sell everything from soap to automobiles. Everything! But it is the wrong kind of sex. Sex in marriage between two believers is an ecstasy and a joy and a peace and a thrill – I feel sorry for some of you who don't know Christ as your Lord and savior. You think you are having a good time, but you're not!

A fourfold protection is promised for those who refrain from adultery: 'First, to protect your marriage . . . Second, to protect your body. Third, to protect you psychologically. Fourth, to protect society.'

Graham condemns the unrepentant: 'These are totally depraved people. Their consciences are either dead or seared. And for some of them, it may already be too late.' For teenagers, he promises 'victory over sex' with Christ. For older sinners, 'Christ can forgive the past . . . What a wonderful thing to be totally cleansed!'

On the last page of the article, the same young couple have changed into jeans and are standing in the window frame of a decaying clapboard house. She is clinging to his arm and he is grimly gazing at the horizon. The suggestion is they have decided to marry and are building their nest in the midst of a collapsing society. Graham wraps up his article with an AIDS-as-sin metaphor: 'We all have a disease worse than AIDS, and that disease is called sin. We are all infected, and we all need to be cleansed by the Great Physician. The Great Physician is the Lord Jesus Christ.'

Jimmy Swaggart Ministries

Born in 1935 in Baton Rouge, Louisiana, Jimmy Swaggart is an ordained minister of the Assemblies of God. This Pentacostal church, established in 1914, anticipates the imminent coming of Christ and consequently rejects the social order and emphasizes spiritual gifts, especially healing through prayer and speaking in tongues. The congregation of this church, as well as Swaggart's viewers, tend to be blue-collar workers who agree with the Christian Right and find their identity expressed in the bluegrass country and western songs performed by Swaggart and his cousin, Jerry Lee Lewis. As a televangelist, Swaggart's outreach extends far beyond the boundaries of his denomination, and his personal wealth places him in a different social stratum than his audience. Nevertheless, he is loyal to the aims of the Assemblies of God and preaches a radical separation from the world and its temptations. These temptations include movies, dancing, drinking, smoking, and pornography. He condemns abortion and divorce and has been known to make statements that offend Catholics, Jews, feminists, and gays of both sexes (Melton, 1989; Lippy, 1989).

Jimmy Swaggart's views on AIDS are expressed in an article that appeared in *The Evangelist* in 1987, and was enclosed in a letter sent to me by Swaggart's administrative assistant, dated 6 November 1987. The article is entitled, 'Is AIDS a Judgment from God?' Swaggart replies, 'No, AIDS is not a plague sent by God, [it] is a result of the evil, wicked, profligate lifestyle of the homosexual community.' The evangelist then claims AIDS 'had its beginning in' or 'originated with the homosexual community,' so that every baby, every innocent individual contracting the disease 'can thank the homosexual community for his death.'

Swaggart goes on to provide an excellent illustration of what Berger would see as the 'homosexual panic' arising from the denial of society's sexual program (Berger, 1969:24):

The sin of homosexuality is one of the most filthy, rotten, degenerate, degrading, hellish lifestyles that's ever been incorporated into the human family. Its birth is in hell . . . it is a direct affront to the human race . . . It is also the worst insult to God ever conceived of by Hell.

Swaggart's advice to his congregation is to pray for a cure from the scientific community because, although 'God can cure . . . few healings will result from this terrible disease.' Unstricken homosexuals should 'ask God to give [them] a wife and prepare to live for the Lord Jesus Christ. The stricken ones 'can only ask God to have mercy . . . and prepare to meet God.'

The Church of Jesus Christ, Scientist

Christian Science's position on AIDS rejects the notion of divine judgment or punishment for sin and stresses the need for compassion and spiritual healing. Mary Baker Eddy rebelled even as a child against the stark Calvinistic view of God as foredooming a major portion of the human race to eternal damnation. In *Science and Health* she states clearly: 'No final judgment awaits mortals, for the judgment day of wisdom comes hourly and continually, even the judgment by which mortal man is divested of all material error' (Eddy, 1934:291).

Consistent with this position, the *Christian Science Monitor* (26 March 1990) asserts: 'We've come a long way since the old theological view that envisioned God as a largely harsh judge handing out sentences to hell for deviations from His Law.' Mrs Eddy's view of the millennium is that a new heaven and a new earth cannot be terrestrial or material, but must be spiritual. Moreover, she rejects the Second Coming as a literal historical event but emphasizes salvation as a present experience rather than as a future possession: 'Now,' cried the apostle, 'is the accepted time: behold, now is the day of salvation' (Eddy, 1934:39). Christian Science, then, might be more accurately categorized as amillennial. The church's refusal to separate the goats from the lambs, and their repudiation of the public's tendency to condemn PWAs, appears to stem from their founder's teaching that sin is an illusion (albeit a persistent and powerful one) that is not banished even by the 'change called death.' Their statement on the church's perspective, which was originally written for an AIDS ministry surveying religious communities, is a call for compassion. It also implies a critical view of society's lack of compassion and perhaps of the judgmental attitudes towards PWAs of other Christian churches. The challenge that Christian Scientists choose to confront in AIDS is to avoid 'the fatal beliefs that error is as real as Truth, that evil is equal in power to good, if not superior, and that discord is as normal as harmony . . .' (quoted in *The Christian Science Monitor* 92:13). Thus Christian Scientists express their intention of solving the problem of AIDS through renewing their faith in the power of God's love, and of redoubling their efforts to heal those afflicted.

> We won't be immobilized by disaster, but through spiritual affection and understanding we'll find the truth that does direct humanity toward divine Life and Love . . . Like the Samaritan, we'll find a way to bind up the wounds and play a significant role in the re-emergence of genuine spiritual healing. (*Christian Science Monitor*, 26 March 1990)

In an editorial addressed to fellow Christian Scientists, Allison W. Phinney of the *Christian Science Sentinel* (11 April 1988) notes that doctors 'fear that a cure cannot be found' and calls for more practical efforts to heal, rather than for more talk about healing, since the medical establishment has failed: 'Plainly, it isn't true that a medical knowledge grounded in materialism has all the answers mankind will ever need.' In fact, 'the world desperately needs to learn more now about the definite, lawful, potent nature of spiritual healing.' Whereas doctors and scientists are ineffective in combating AIDS, Phinney states that, for Christian Scientists, 'no disease is what it seems': 'If one malady seems to be more resistant to healing than another, it is not actually the disease that is resistant, but the human concept producing the disease.' The most striking feature of AIDS, immune deficiency, is remarked upon to strengthen Christian Scientists beliefs on healing and to encourage their healers: 'medical researchers are beginning to realize how strongly the immune function of the human body is increased by unselfish love.'

The final message in this editorial is a call for action: 'The world needs this spiritual experience. It is crying out for healing as never before.'

On the evidence of a letter written to me by Nathan Talbot, Head of Publishing, Boston, Christian Science practitioners have been active in attempting to heal people with AIDS. Since Christian Scientists would be reluctant to go to doctors for blood tests, presumably these healers must be devoting their efforts to patients outside the church. Talbot asserts, 'There have been healings of AIDS in Christian Science' (Talbot, personal communication, 5 February 1990). When I wrote back asking for more detail, he responded, 'For the reason mentioned in that letter, we haven't sought to obtain names or details on specific healings of AIDS and are reluctant to subject any individuals healed to the weight of public scepticism until they decide for themselves to speak about their experience.'

The Church of the Latter-Day Saints

The Mormon church was founded in 1830 in Palmyra, New York, by the Prophet Joseph Smith. In 1843 he announced his revelation on plural and celestial marriage: if performed in the temples under the authority of the priesthood, marriage will continue 'for time and eternity' and family life will be resumed in the celestial kingdom. Foster notes that this revelation raised marriage to a position of supreme importance as the only means by which salvation of body and spirit could be achieved:

> In heaven, men who had contracted such marriages would be great patriarchs having 'all power,' surrounded by their own families . . . [they] would eventually move on to rule over whole new worlds in conjunction with their wives . . . (Foster, 1981:145)

Polygamy, which was practised until the 1890s, was believed to be a particularly exalted form of celestial marriage.

The Mormon church espouses a premillennialist's view of history, but in the one article appearing in the *Ensign* that mentions

AIDS there is no attempt to work the 'new plague' into the Mormon version of the Second Coming or the Day of Judgment. Instead, President Gordon B. Hinckley takes this opportunity to affirm the importance and divinely ordained nature of the Latter-Day Saints' code of sexual morality:

> There is a plague of fearsome dimensions moving across the world ... We ... hope that discoveries will make possible both prevention and healing ... But regardless of such discoveries, the observance of one ... divinely given rule would do more than all else to check this epidemic. That is chastity before marriage and fidelity after marriage. Prophets of God have repeatedly taught through the ages that practices of homosexual relations, fornication and adultery are grievous sins. (Hinckley, 1987:46–7)

This leader is the first counsellor in the First Presidency, which consists of three men who provide spiritual and moral guidance to over four million Latter-Day Saints in the United States and Canada. In his statement the importance of marriage and its sacred character are emphasized:

> The Lord has proclaimed that marriage between a man and a woman is ordained of God and is intended to be an eternal relationship bounded by trust, and fidelity. Latter-Day Saints, of all people, should marry with this sacred objective in mind.

President Hinckley identifies the two major vulnerable areas for the Mormon community: its teenagers and its rapid influx of new converts who are eligible for temple marriage after one full year of celibacy and living according to the Word of Wisdom. He quotes historians Will and Ariel Durant:

> A youth boiling with hormones will wonder why he should not give full freedom to his sexual desires; and if he is unchecked by customs, morals or laws, he may ruin his life before he matures sufficiently to understand that sex is a river of fire that must be banked and

cooled by a hundred restraints before it is not to consume in chaos both the individual and the group. (Durant & Durant, 1968:35–6)

Hinckley is uncompromising on the issue of homosexuality:

Marriage should not be viewed as a therapeutic step to solve problems such as homosexual inclinations or practices, which first should clearly be overcome with a firm and fixed determination not to slip into such practices again.

The church's strictures on sex education are defended. Since the state of Utah has prohibited sex education in school without parental consent, and the Attorney-General has even forbidden the use of the words 'condom' and 'intercourse' in public schools, the church had been under pressure, from U.S. Surgeon General C. Everett Koop and the AIDS Project Utah, to change its policy ('Heartache in Happy Valley,' 1988). President Hinckley is possibly responding to this pressure when he states:

More sex education in public schools will not reverse the damaging legacy of the sexual revolution unless the clear message is premarital chastity and marital monogamy ... Sex education fights the modesty and morality endemic to human life. (Hinckley, 1987:47)

While emphasizing that adherence to Latter-Day Saints' standards of sexual behaviour will protect the individual and 'check the epidemic,' Hinckley nevertheless counsels members to have compassion for PWAs:

Having said this, I desire now to say with emphasis that our concern for the bitter fruit of sin is coupled with Christlike sympathy for its victims, innocent or culpable. We advocate the example of our Lord who condemned sin, yet loved the sinner. We should reach out with kindness and comfort to the afflicted, ministering to their needs and assisting them with their problems. (Hinckley, 1987:47)

The Jehovah's Witnesses

The Watchtower and Bible Tract Society devoted the 22 April 1986 issue of their magazine, *Awake!*, to the AIDS problem. While there is no attempt to work the AIDS symbol into their apocalyptic theory, the Witnesses do use it to underscore their standards of sexual behaviour. Besides outlawing sexual relationships before or outside marriage, Witnesses must observe other rules of sexual conduct: 'The Witnesses are specifically forbidden to masturbate, laugh at dirty jokes, . . . go out on a date without a chaperone . . . give rein to unbridled passion while having sexual intercourse' (White, 1967:84).

For Witnesses, the AIDS threat serves as a reminder that their sexual program is divinely ordained:

> Yet is more than a biological fact – morality is involved. The moral standards that society has chosen to flout did not originate with humans. A superior intelligence had them recorded long ago. ('AIDS: Who Are at Risk,' 1986:8)

The Jehovah Witnesses' position on blood transfusions is well known, and the fact that AIDS can be transmitted through blood is used to reinforce their position:

> First, avoid the sources of contamination . . . by living in harmony with the standards of conduct that Almighty God provided. Consider how these would have protected thousands now dying of AIDS . . . Significantly, the Bible forbade humans to consume blood. It says: '. . . keep abstaining from blood' – Acts 15:28, 29. ('AIDS: Who Are at Risk,' 1986:8)

The article points out that homosexuals are 'the most susceptible group,' then quotes from the New English Bible: 'Make no mistake . . . none who are guilty of adultery or of homosexual perversion . . . will possess the kingdom of God' (Corinthians 6:9).

As a comment on another susceptible group, heterosexuals with multiple sexual partners, the following biblical passages are quoted:

> Let marriage be honourable among all . . . for God will judge forni-
> cators and adulterers. – Hebrews 13:4. Deaden, therefore, your body
> members that are upon earth as respects fornication, uncleanness,
> sexual appetite . . . On account of these things the wrath of God is
> coming. – Colossians 3:5,6.

The April 1988 issue of *Awake!* features the article, 'Are We in the Last Days?' which argues that the war, famine, and plague afflicting the world today are the fulfilment of biblical prophecy, and cites as an example Jesus' warning that one of the signs of the Last Days would be 'pestilences' (Luke 21:11). AIDS, cancer, and heart disease are mentioned. The death of millions from these diseases is evidence for 'the pale horse of death and deadly plague, the fourth horse of the apocalypse' ('Are We in the Last Days,' 1988:11).

Although it is not stated overtly, in both articles the implication is that AIDS is not a problem for Jehovah's faithful servants, but is rather a visible sign of those who 'fall short of perfection in their behaviour' and who, in the millennium, will be 'consigned to eternal oblivion from which there will be no release' (Beckford, 1975:6).

The Seventh-Day Adventists

One hundred forty years have passed since William Miller and his followers' 'Great Disappointment' of 1844, and the last decade has been one of turmoil for church leaders coping with the unexpectedly long delay of the advent. On the one hand there has been a call to restore primitive adventism and 'preserve the landmarks' of Ellen G. White's vision. On the other hand, a new generation of Adventists believe they must seek their own 'present truth' and urge church members to foster a stronger community through a clearer separation between church and state, and through removing inequalities between the sexes, among the races, and between the clergy and the laity. The Adventists have a history of long, complex debates over such controversial issues as birth control, abortion, divorce, race relations, and homosexuality. While providing a forum for open discussion and dissent, the church has remained conservative in its orientation while avoiding public statements might antagonize or alienate its more liberal and youthful members (Pearson, 1990). Therefore, Adventist views on AIDS must be understood as reflecting the ongoing tension between traditional values and the search for contemporary relevance that distinguishes the church today.

The *Adventist Review* of 24 July 1986 features an editorial entitled 'AIDS: An Adventist Perspective.' It explicitly states that AIDS is *not* a sign of God's wrath ('We shouldn't look upon people with AIDS as coming under the direct judgment of God'), and that PWAs do not deserve the disease any more than an Adventist who gets sick because he does not exercise or who 'pours on the salt and sugar.' For Adventists, the important issue and moral stance in respect to AIDS lies in the treatment of its victims:

If Jesus were here today, how would he treat people with AIDS?

Victims of AIDS are the lepers of our society. We know how Jesus treated the lepers of His day.

We cannot bring healing to these modern lepers, but we should receive them in the spirit of Jesus. Although in many cases they are suffering as the result of their own actions, their offense is ultimately no worse than the respectable sins we indulge in ... Their human condition, in current medical terms, is hopeless; but Jesus is their hope.

At present, Adventist hospitals are treating patients with AIDS ... The church, now hardly touched by the AIDS epidemic, will feel its impact. How we react to people with AIDS will reveal the genuineness of our Christianity. ('AIDS: An Adventist Perspective,' 1986:5)

The *Adventist Review* cautions: 'We shouldn't be part of the panic over AIDS, and urges 'Christian ministers [to] reach out ... in support of AIDS victims and their families.' While careful to avoid any homophobic comments, another Adventist writer uses the AIDS threat to reinforce Adventist standards of sexual behaviour:

> Christians have long advocated the limitation of sexual intercourse to the marriage relationship and encouraged premarital abstinence ... Now is the time to reinforce the idea that God gave His moral law as a means of protection for His children. (*Ministry*, September 1986:23)

Of all the churches in this study, the Adventists appear the least worried about contagion. Their literature states that PWAs not be assigned separate pews in church and suggests the following guidelines for those caring for PWAs at home:

> An automatic dishwasher is adequate for cleaning dishes ... A patient may share the bathroom with other members of the family. Visibly soiled facilities should be cleaned ... Never share toothbrushes [or] razor blades when there is a possibility of a transfer of blood. (*Ministry*, September 1986:23)

In summary, the Adventists' position on AIDS does not diverge very far from that of the American upper-middle class, as expressed in the many articles on the topic appearing in the *New York Times* over the last few years. The Adventists' refusal to fit AIDS into their premillennial theory, and their reasonable, 'let's keep informed' attitude is perhaps due to their assimilation of American middle-class values and deferred-reward thinking, described by Gary Schwartz:

> It promises success in this world and in the kingdom shortly to come to those who honor God's commands punctiliously. It equates the practical virtues which enhance one's chances for upward social mobility with the characteristics of God's elect, insuring that those who take God's stern warning seriously will also strive to prove they belong to this highly favored group. (Schwartz, 1970:212)

AIDS and Christian Apocalypticism

There are some major differences in the part AIDS plays within the eschatological dramas of the televangelists and the Christian sects featured in this chapter. These differences, and the degree of prominence awarded to the virus within their apocalyptic theory, are best understood by referring to William Martin's and Andrew Weigert's outlines of the different strains of millennial theory in America.

Historians have traditionally divided American antebellum religions into two categories, which are distinguished by their beliefs concerning Christ's Second Coming: premillennialists claim He will usher in a thousand years of peace, and postmillennialists claim He will return after the thousand-year period to judge the living and the dead. Since the variety and complexity of apocalyptic theory in millenarian movements is overwhelming, a simpler method of classification is used here: those groups that hold out no hope for this world and tend to regard society as evil and corrupt, richly deserving its impending destruction, are termed *premillennialists*, and those groups that believe the world is on the threshold of unparalleled improvement are termed *postmillennialists*.

As Table 1 (p. 40) demonstrates, six of the churches in this study espouse a premillennialist philosophy, one falls in the postmillennialist, and one in the amillennialist category. The most widespread premillennial theory is that developed by John Nelson Darby and published in the 1909 Scofield Reference Bible. In his scheme, 'the triggering action will be the Rapture' (Martin, 1982:32) in which the faithful will be caught up to heaven. Then will follow seven years of tribulation, which will include plagues and pestilences. The False Prophet will then ally with the Antichrist and wage war against Christ who will win the Battle of Armageddon, at which point the saints will enter the millennium, 'an age characterized by good weather, peace, and end to crime' (Martin, 1982:32). Christian fundamentalists and TV evangelists adhere to this model and tend to share the view that any sign of deterioration in the nation's economic, political, or moral health foreshadows

TABLE 1
AIDS and Religious Organizations

Religious Organization	Type of Millennialism	End of World?	Homosexuals Deserve AIDS?	Victims Excluded?	Monogamy Solution?	Inferior Consciousness?
Jimmy Swaggert Ministries	premillennial	no	yes	no	yes	no
Worldwide Church of God (Church of Tomorrow)	premillennial	yes	yes	–	yes	no
Jehovah's Witnesses	postmillennial	yes	yes	yes	yes	no
Seventh-Day Adventists	premillennial	no	no	no	yes	no
Christian Scientists	amillennial	no	no	no	yes	yes
Latter-Day Saints	premillennial	no	no	no	yes	no

the Second Coming. Hence, as Martin points out, 'almost any scrap of truly bad news is hailed as another sign that we are in the homestretch of history,' and is even greeted with 'an odd sort of self-conscious optimism' (Martin, 1982:34). Graham, Armstrong, Adams, and Swaggart adhere to this model, which Weigert (1988) terms 'fundamentalist eschatology,' and their responses to AIDS are consistent with this type, which Weigert contrasts with the ideal of 'liberal eschatology.' Their lack of interest in a possible cure or medically approved methods of stemming the epidemic are the logical outcome of their belief in God's unchangeable plan, the imminence of Endtime, and their confidence in being 'born again' – since a personal decision to accept Jesus will guarantee their rapture to a safe place while nuclear war and plagues cleanse the earth.

Swaggart's insistence that AIDS is not sent by God, but is rather of Satanic origin, spread by demonic hordes of homosexuals, reflects the dualistic world view of dispensationalists who perceive current events in terms of a battle between good and evil. His role as a healer perhaps inclines him to share the view of the early Christians, for whom illness was the torture of demons which God's healing power could allay (White, 1965:291–4).

The Armstrong brand of pietism is rather different from the other two evangelists. The WWCG reject the born-again plan of salvation, and instead base their eligibility for rapture on their identity as Anglo-Israelites, which is justified through their commitment to the church and its rules. Thus, *The Plain Truth* demonstrates at least some concern over protecting the family unit and the congregation from the AIDS virus, in contrast to Adams and Swaggart, who emphasize individual salvation. As Weigert notes, 'The supernatural frame of Fundamentalist eschatology provides an identity and vocabulary of motive for making sense out of issues like being eternally happy while separated from unconverted family and friends' (Weigert, 1988).

The two older premillennialist churches espouse a different eschatological model which is rooted in British and American evangelicism and Methodism of the Victorian era. The Latter-Day Saints and Seventh-Day Adventists, while holding to their beliefs in the

Second Coming and the millennium at some unspecified time in the future, have been influenced by liberal eschatology. This 'starts with the present and tries to work towards a future inspired by Christ's message but empirically unknowable.' It rejects 'literal End Time thinking' and 'interprets eschatology as a promise and mission to develop God's Kingdom on earth' (Weigert, 1988:184). Both churches have assimilated the eighteenth-century Enlightenment idea of progress as secularized eschatology, and thus hope science will find a cure for the virus. They reject the pessimism and determinism of Calvinism and insist on the individual's control over personal salvation; that through hard work and self-control one can earn a place in the eternal kingdom. They are optimistic in the sense that they reject the notion of eternal damnation, representing a shift from Christ-centred eschatology to a human-centred responsibility. The moral significance of AIDS is not divine punishment, therefore, but rather a call to exercise compassion and charity. This response is consistent with Weigert's 'liberal' Christian, whose interpretation of prophecy is analogical, 'calling humans to act morally for the good of all' (Weigert, 1988:184).

The Jehovah's Witnesses can be classified as postmillennialists, since they believe that Christ's coming has already taken place (albeit invisibly) in 1974 in order to gather 140,000 co-rulers for the Kingdom of God. The Battle of Armageddon is projected far into the future, however, so that the intervening period allows time for evangelical activity and the gradual moral perfecting of individuals. Thus the Witnesses hold a 'gradualist view of history and a relatively optimistic conception of the future' typical of postmillennialists (Beckford, 1975:201). Past experience with prophetic disconfirmation, and an uncharismatic leadership today, would account for the relative caution (compared to the WWCG or Adams) with which they embark on their doomsday extrapolations of the 'new plague.' Rather than seeing it as a new sign of divine disapproval, they list it as one of the signs of the Last Days and a visible branding of those who, owing to their immoral behaviour, will be consigned to everlasting oblivion.

In many of these small Christian churches, their philosophies of sexuality are inextricably linked to their apocalyptic expectations and their eschatologies. Adventists in their literal reading of Genesis do not doubt that homosexuality is a perversion of God's ideal for human relationships. Their notion of 'sanctification' – that each believer grows in virtue until a perfect church is formed, ready to receive the Second Coming – necessarily includes marriage and parenting and excludes alternative sexual lifestyles. For Latter-Day Saints, marriage is eternal and procreation is a means of ushering in the waiting spirits and hastening the end of time. The sexual mores of Jehovah's Witnesses and Armstrong followers are also taught as divinely ordained. AIDS, which is associated with homosexuality and non-procreative and extramarital sex, has become a symbol of the profane love that preoccupies those sinners beyond the walls of the sect and lures them away from the narrow path of righteousness.

THREE

Isolating Utopias

*The Rajneesh/Osho Movement, The Unification Church, The
International Society for Krishna Consciousness, The Messianic
Communities, The Children of God/The Family, The Politics
of Isolation*

The history of heresy in America is a landscape studded with
utopian communes. New spiritual marriages and eugenics programs were ongoing experiments in nineteenth-century 'cities on
a hill' such as those of the Shakers and Oneida Perfectionists, and
were often part of their preparations for world's end. Sheltered
under the authoritarian wings of home-grown messiahs, committed communitarians sought to create a New Adam, free of original
sin, who might enjoy perfect health and anticipate immortality in
the predicted meeting of Heaven and Earth. These frontier prophets expounded tautologies of purity, creating elaborate body rituals
to facilitate the transformation of their followers from *Homo sapiens*
to *Homo superiorus*.

Communal and millenarian movements today exhibit similar
patterns and preoccupations. Unconsciously imitating their cult
forebearers in practising celibacy, free love, or polygamy, many
contemporary utopians have resumed the age-old quest for what
Mormon historian Klaus J. Hansen dubbed 'sexual solutions to the
problem of death.' All the groups in this chapter propose spiritual
strategies for coping with sex and death that express their eschatological expectations and have constructed new symbologies for
the human body. They have designed taboos governing food, diet,
and hygiene to repel or neutralize what they perceive as the polluting influences of the secular world. Sexual energy is rechannel-
led and the exits and entrances of the human body are guarded,
thereby fortifying the boundaries of their communities.

The statements on AIDS issuing from the communal groups reveal a deep intolerance for sexual and social disorder – and a strong concern for protecting their social boundaries. Thus, solutions to the AIDS epidemic adopted by totalistic new religions are generally more extreme and decisive than those recommended by Christian churches. Precautionary measures advised by their leaders tend to be rigorously imposed, with very little left to the discretion of the individual. Unlike the churches, whose concern is to protect the biological family or the congregation, these groups are concerned with guarding the circumference of the 'spiritual family.'

Perhaps because they inhabit contested territory at the margins of American religious life – or because of their sectarian stance, their spiritual 'outsidership' – these religions perceive AIDS as a threat that is at once microbiological and moral. Unlike the older Christian minorities (Mormons, Christian Scientists, Jehovah's Witnesses) who attend Sunday services in respectably dressed family groups, and can therefore pass as denominations, new religions are perceived as deviant and controversial. Already stigmatized as 'cults,' struggling to correct media stereotypes of fanatical leaders and ranks of 'brainwashed zombies,' these groups cannot afford to welcome people into their midst who bear an even greater social stigma.

Hence, new religious policies towards AIDS and its carriers express a need to fortify the boundaries of small societies against what they perceive as the profane and hostile host society surrounding them. For this reason, they often adopt the isolating response to AIDS.

The Rajneesh Movement (Friends of Osho)

The new religious movement that grew out of the popular discourses of an Indian-born philosophy professor, Bhagwan Shree Rajneesh, has instituted the most rigorous precautions against AIDS, and exhibits the most elaborate metaphorical thinking about the disease of all the groups in this study.[2] Rajneesh, throughout his career as a spiritual master, had occasionally dropped hints concerning disasters of a nuclear, geological, or environmental nature, but when he emerged from three-and-a-half years of silence in 1984, he announced with greater precision than usual that two-thirds of humanity would die of the disease by the end of the century. He quoted from Nostradamus' *The Centuries* and claimed that his red-garbed *sannyasins* or disciples would be among the survivors to build a new society based on meditative consciousness and ruled by women. Shortly after this event the Rajneesh Medical Corporation at Rajneeshpuram (the group's utopian city in Oregon) instituted various precautionary measures to protect the community: couples were obliged to wear condoms and rubber gloves during sexual intercourse and to refrain from kissing. Elaborate procedures for the preparation of food and waste disposal were introduced: cooks wore latex gloves, dishes were rinsed in bleach, and doorknobs and telephone receivers were sprayed daily with alcohol. Birthday candles were not blown out, but clapped out (Palmer, 1986; Fitzgerald, 1986). 'Super Sex Kits' containing condoms, latex gloves, Koromex jelly, and an information brochure were advertised in the *Rajneesh Times* and sold in Rajneesh centres.

Rajneesh's statements concerning AIDS illustrate Sontag's ideas (1978) on illness as symbols of social disorder and inferior consciousness. She points out that tuberculosis was once thought to be a pathology of the will. Rajneesh associates AIDS with a loss of will:

> Humanity is losing its will to live. If the mind loses the will to live it will be affected in the body by the dropping of resistance against sickness, against death. If the will to live disappears, the sex will be the most vulnerable area of life to invite death. As it appears to me, the disease is spiritual. (*Rajneesh Times*, 18 January 1985)

Like the other church leaders in this study, Rajneesh uses the AIDS threat to emphasize the sacred quality of his movement's sexual program, and by defining homosexual behaviour as profane, or 'against nature,' he is asserting that Rajneeshee heterosexual relationships – which are deviant by mainstream standards –

reflect a 'right' relationship with the sacred cosmos and with Bhagwan Himself:

> AIDS is the ultimate development of homosexuality and it has no cure. You have gone so far away from Nature that there is no way back. You have broken all the bridges behind you: that is the disease AIDS. (*Rajneesh Times*, 16 August 1985)

In a discourse reported in the *Rajneesh Times International* (1 March 1988), Rajneesh blames organized religion for creating homosexuality by segregating the sexes and enforcing celibacy which, in turn, generated the virus:

> Homosexuals – because they were perverted – created the disease AIDS. Heterosexuality creates life, life for your children and a divine life for you. Homosexuality is absolutely barren. It does not create anything.

Rajneesh accused the Vatican and the Pope for bringing about, if indirectly, the AIDS plague:

> The Vatican is the most responsible for creating AIDS. And the Pope has to be termed, not as a representative of God but as a superintendent of an AIDS hospital ... The name of the Vatican should be changed: AIDS-Camp seems to be perfectly good.

(Aside from its obvious shock value, this statement could be interpreted as expressing a sense of marginality, and a desire to strengthen the boundaries between his community and the outside world, which is regarded as a source of chaos and pollution.)

Rajneesh, unlike the other leaders quoted in this study, suggests that AIDS is caused, not by too much licence, but by repression. In this way he resembles Wilhelm Reich who described cancer as 'the stagnation of the flow of the life energy of the organism,' thereby contributing to the mystique surrounding cancer as a 'disease of insufficient passion afflicting those who are sexually repressed, inhibited, unspontaneous, incapable of expressing anger' (Sontag,

1978:21). Rajneesh suggests in the passage below that AIDS is the outcome of society's repression of the individual's emotions and desires, and recommends cutting ties with the past and adopting a *carpe diem* attitude as a protection against the disease:

> Man is becoming mature, aware that he has been cheated by the priests, by the parents, by the pedagogues; he has been simply cheated by everyone, and they have been feeding him false hopes. The day he matures and realizes this, the desire to live falls apart, and the first thing to be wounded by it will be your sexuality. To me, that is AIDS.
>
> I am simply trying to teach you to live without your will, to live joyously. It is the tomorrow that goes on poisoning. Forget the yesterdays, the tomorrows. This is our day. Just by being fully alive in it is such a power that not only you can live, you can make others aflame, afire.
>
> If you are involved in the herenow, you are so completely out of the area where infection is possible. AIDS is to me an existential sickness. Only meditation can help. Only meditation can release your energy herenow. (*Rajneesh Times*, 18 January 1985)

AIDS tests are compulsory for devotees of Bhagwan Shree Rajneesh. The *Rajneesh Times* of 13 September 1985 reports that the whole community at Rajneeshpuram, in Oregon, were tested. Rajneeshpuram, founded in 1981, was disbanded in 1985–6; Rajneesh returned to his former ashram in Poona, India, and adopted the new title 'Osho,' or 'teacher of meditation' (Japanese). It became a non-negotiable regulation that all *sannyasins* undergo an AIDS test every three months. The Montreal *Grada Rajneesh* newsletter of February 1987 announced:

> all visitors to Rajneeshdam Neo-sannyas Commune in Poona will be required to bring a doctor's certificate – not more than three months old – showing the results of a recent AIDS test. Those whose tests show a positive result are requested not to come.

A local leader in the Osho community, Ma Jivan Mada, described

how very thorough the AIDS precautions in Rajneeshpuram actually were:[3]

> Our dishes went through a triple wash, after being washed with
> soapy water and rinsed, they went through a clorox bath in propor-
> tions of 15 drops of clorox per gallon of water. In the residential
> kitchens one more step was added, all the used cups and dishes were
> first collected in a special 'clorox bath' container, and were washed
> afterwards in the 'three-step' wash. In every toilet appeared an al-
> cohol spray bottle and everyone was asked to alcohol their hands
> after having washed them first with soap and water, then, to spray
> the faucets with alcohol before leaving the bathroom. It was really
> beautiful to see, how everyone devotedly followed these steps. I
> even remember how many of us carried our own little alcohol bottles
> everywhere we went. As far as the cleaning of our bathrooms, show-
> ers and toilets, they were cleaned twice a day and disinfected, sur-
> faces sprayed with alcohol, floors mopped with clorox solution. As
> for the food and cooking areas, they were naturally being handled
> with gloves. Gloves were used also for working on the farm and for
> picking vegetables. Before putting on the gloves we used to wash
> our hands with soap and water, then alcohol them, and, at the end
> of the day, the gloves went through a 'triple wash' and were hung
> to dry until the next day.
>
> During meals, before we could go through the food line to take
> our food, we used to spray our hands with alcohol. No food was
> touched with bare hands, tongs were amply available, and the tables
> were already sprayed with alcohol before we sat at them.

She also listed rules issued by the Rajneesh Medical Corporation
to the Rajneeshpuram residents, which appeared on signs hung
up in the Hotel Rajneesh:

> *Do not share cigarettes, eating utensils, or any items that have touched*
> *your mouth.*
>
> *Break candy bars in the same wrapper so each person can take a piece while*
> *not touching other pieces.*

Popcorn should be poured into each person's hand.

Do not lick pages of a book or journal to turn them.

Do not lick thread to thread a needle.

Use a moistened sponge to seal envelopes.

Both the handle and mouthpiece of telephones should be cleaned with alcohol after each use.

Use individual toothpaste, individual toiletries and deodorant.

Never share a towel. Each towel should be used only once and then washed.

Avoid sexual intercourse during the woman's period.

Take showers before and after sexual intercourse.

Be sure that no one goes into the lake with an open cut or infection or when menstruating.

Cleanse your genitals before going into the lake or the river, and use a second wipe to clean your hands.

Mada described how visitors and those who tested HIV positive were treated:

> Visitors, upon arrival at Rajneeshpuram . . . were shown a video prepared by the crew. Made with humor and taste, it beautifully illustrated all the AIDS precautions described above.
>
> One of Osho's major guidances to prevent the AIDS epidemic from spreading is – compulsory testing and segregation of the AIDS victims.
>
> They can move to a special campus near every big city . . . There are doctors who are suffering from AIDS, these doctors should be moved to those campuses. We can prevent the rest of humanity being affected, and without destroying the dignity of the people who are suffering from AIDS. It is so simple, and they can work, they can do whatsoever they are skilled in: but they should remain in their own monastery.

She notes that the ashram now demands more frequent AIDS testing in response to a worsening world situation:

These drastic measures of compulsory testing and segregating communities implemented by Osho might appear inhuman and undemocratic, but if one looks deeper, *it is the only way to save unnecessary wastage of lives.* It is no longer a question of democracy, but of LIFE and DEATH.

The Osho Commune International is the ONLY AIDS-FREE ZONE in the WORLD TODAY. When Osho moved back to Poona in 1987, where naturally thousands of his disciples followed, one of the prerequisites to enter the ashram, in order to participate in meditations, therapy groups, and attend Osho's twice daily discourses, was an HIV test of less than six months old.

In 1989, in view of the increasing incidence of AIDS in India, the commune took further precautions by requiring a negative HIV test of less than three months old. Today, because of the recent explosion in AIDS cases world-wide, a negative test of less than one month old is required.

The ashram authorities have made arrangements with the local hospital where, thanks to the latest HIV testing methods, an AIDS test result can be obtained within one or two hours. Today, before you can enter the ashram, a gate pass is issued with your photograph and an expiration date of your AIDS test which you must present each time you enter the 'gateless gate' of the ashram.

Mada finds a certain prophetic wisdom in Osho's early advice on the AIDS crisis:

As Osho suggested in 1984: 'If you are ready and can drop sex altogether through your understanding and without repression, this is the safest protection from the disease. Or remain with the same partner, merge into the same partner, move more and more into intimacy and less into sexual activity ... The time has come for the sexual habits and the sexual carelessness of the modern age to end.'

She adds, 'One of the most popular sayings amongst *sannyasins* today is, 'I am really not interested in sex, all I would like to do is lay [*sic*] down beside you and feel your energy.'

Mada recommends that Osho's AIDS policies, although criticized, should be adopted as a paradigm for the rest of society:

It is ironic, that having been widely condemned and internationally criticized as a 'sex guru,' and his disciples falsely advertised as perverts and drug addicts, the Osho Commune International is the cleanest, safest, most beautiful and loving place on earth today.

A very different perspective on Rajneeshpuram's AIDS prevention procedures appeared in a story featured in the *Rajneesh Times* on 27 September 1985, which might be a warning of the dystopian possibilities of compulsory AIDS testing. In this article, one Ma Anand Zeno, a resident of Rajneeshpuram, relates how she was tested with the whole community of disciples on 13 September 1985, but was falsely informed by the head nurse, Puja, that she had tested positive for AIDS antibodies and must go into total isolation in Desiderata Canyon. She describes her several months in the clinic with a group of men, also with putative compromised immune systems:

Puja ran frantically around, spraying alchohol over everything . . . with a wry smile and a saccharine line saying, 'This is a beautiful opportunity for you to go into the meditation of death' On the rare occasions we were visited, visitors wore surgical masks, gloves and gowns, keeping a distance from us, implying that we were physically and psychologically untouchable . . . it was actually seven weeks before I was retested. And then, the ominous silence . . . finally, two weeks later, I received the message that the test results were unclear and I would have to be retested.

Zeno describes her segregation from the commune:

And it was another planet. The only contact we had . . . was during morning discourse. We came late, sat by ourselves, and were cautioned against talking too closely with other people (the contagion of spit) . . . Every avenue of communication was blocked with the constant reminders that in every way I was endangering the community if I touched anything or anyone.

Zeno reports how she was fed drugs and began to develop symptoms of the disease: 'I began to have muscle aches, headaches and cramps that would come and go.' She found her fellow prisoners were experiencing similar symptoms they interpreted as AIDS, but she began to ask, 'Why was it that the attendants were given strict instructions to never eat or drink in our trailer? Why had such explicit directions been given about who was to occupy which room?' The motive behind Zeno's incarceration was explained by a former resident as follows: Zeno's work or 'worship' in the commune was with audio-visual equipment, and she had taped a meeting in which Rajneesh had harshly criticized Ma Anand Sheela, who was his personal secretary. When the time came to show the video to the assembled commune, Sheela announced that the equipment had broken down. Zeno had contradicted her, and raised embarrassing questions concerning why this particular tape must not be shown.[4] The other 'patients' in the Desiderata clinic also happened to be dissidents (or homosexuals) during Sheela's reign over the commune in her (self-created) office as 'Chancellor of Rajneeshism.'

Fortunately, Zeno's story has a happy ending. After Sheela and her 'fascist gang' defected, a new core group were elected to run the commune, and the inmates of Desiderata were retested. All but one – a homosexual named Lazarus – received negative results. Zeno expresses her relief and raises some interesting questions concerning the fine line between social responsibility and social control:

> One of the most beautiful things I learned from this experience is how much I love Bhagwan and this commune and each precious moment of the life we live. I feel this community needs to take a new, clear look at the AIDS precautions we have adopted. Do they come out of the paranoia and psychological manipulation of the old regime or are they actually valid? . . . I feel that the entire community has been brainwashed into an extremist position on AIDS . . . I hope

that we can move with intelligence and love to provide the necessary protection and human caring for every member of the commune. (*Rajneesh Times*, 27 September 1985:B4)

The Unification Church

This new religion, founded in 1954 in Korea by Reverend Sun Myung Moon, has to date produced no more than a few paragraphs on AIDS in its literature. Nevertheless, the church has instituted obligatory AIDS testing for its members before they can participate in the Blessing (popularly known as the 'Moonie Mass Marriages'). Reverend Moon announced during the Matching Ceremony (in which he chooses the marriage partners under divine inspiration) held on 27 and 28 March 1987 at the New Yorker Hotel in Manhattan that AIDS was a 'Sign of the Last Days.'

Since Unification theology is concerned with the pollution of blood through sexual relations, it would appear to offer fertile ground for metaphorical thinking about AIDS. In Reverend Moon's theodicy, the Fall of Man was brought about through Eve's sexual relationship with the angel Lucifer, and the subsequent transmission of her fallen state to Adam through their premarital sexual union. For Unificationists, the consequence of the Fall is that we are all children of Satan and not, as was originally planned, of God. An important step towards redemption, or 'Restoration,' is through marriage to one's divinely ordained spouse, in the course of which one's fallen nature is restored through becoming the spiritual child of the Moons, the New Eve and the New Adam.

In spite of their concern over blood lineage, Unificationists may receive blood transfusions. Since, until recently, all members had to observe a minimum of three years of premarital celibacy and three years of postmarital sexual abstinence, they regard their standards of sexual conduct to be an adequate protection against the disease.

In a published sermon, 'Let Us Go Over the Original Boundary' (1 April 1987), Reverend Moon raises the problem of the predicted casualties from AIDS, and asks, 'Does that mean the Moonie population will be reduced too?' He offers his solution: a doctor who

is 'omnipotent . . . has to know everything and be virtually almighty . . . Only God is such a being.' His medicine is love:

> God will say, 'I have that magic panacea medicine to cure all. The
> name of that medicine is true love . . . True love is that kind of
> powerful cure-all and panacea . . . The Unificationist Church is ap-
> plying this particular prescription. One individual came to the
> church in terrible shape. He was sick, full of aches and pains. But . . .
> after a few months he got better and became stronger and stronger.
> I feel sure he will live a long time – maybe to 100 years of age!

This passage appears in the middle of an intensely mystical
sermon on the interconnectedness of all life and the force of love
that moves protons and electrons. Then Moon goes on to contrast
the 'original world' with the fallen world in which 'love shrinks'
and the physical body 'is completely blocked and isolated.' The
work of God, Moon states, 'had been the work of cleansing . . . This
is called restoration.'

The Unificationists' repudiation of homosexuality makes them
inclined to be unsympathetic towards homosexual PWAs. When
asked what would become of these people, eschatologically speaking, one Unificationist replied, 'When they go to the Spirit World,
they're in for a big shock!' Reverend Moon's position on this matter
resembles Augustine's 'natural good':

> It is the most unnatural kind of love. At the time of creation did
> Adam have any other men to love? Then it is in the Principle that
> woman must love a man and a man must love a woman. Homosex-
> uality is unnatural, against God's law of Creation. (*Master Speaks*,
> 4:5)

Robert Duffy, the former President of the Holy Spirit Association
for the Unification of World Christianity in Canada, expressed the
notion that AIDS was the result of flouting Nature, but was optimistic that scientists will discover a positive use for the HIV virus,
since Nature reflects its Creator Who is wholly good:[5]

I think I can say that there is no concept in Unificationism that the

HIV virus is a God-sent plague to destroy immoral practices, but rather it is a phenomenon of Nature . . . unleashed through practices which I would term 'anti-natural.' Through practices against nature, membranes are broken, bodily fluids are released in ways which the body is not designed to facilitate . . . I would say that the Unificationist position stands solidly on a theology of nature, a nature which rooted in a holy expression of God's love.

For Unificationists, then, AIDS is the outcome of an abuse of love in the Garden of Eden and reinforces the church's sexual program that demands a long period of celibacy in preparation for surrendering to Reverend Moon's choice of spouse.

Concerning the future of AIDS, Unificationists are optimistic, on a scientific as well as on an eschatological level. Scientists, Duffy claims, have discovered how the HIV virus can be used to benefit humanity:

That same powerful virus which is able to kill now, could also be turned to the good and be used to cure. There is a considerable body of research that is working on the use of the HIV virus as an invading force into the cell structure that can be used to recode genetic defects which are present in individuals who, for example, have sickle-cell anaemia. The HIV virus can be used to bring in a corrective code genetically. So, that some powerful and natural force can be turned into the good.

Since Unificationists believe the Second Coming is living among us, and hence espouse a postmillennialist view, the world can only get better and better, and everyone – even practising homosexuals – will be eventually 'restored' in the Spirit World. This attitude speaks more of compassion and less of judgment than those of many Christian fundamentalists who would consign all AIDS sufferers to hell.

The International Society for Krishna Consciousness

The International Society for Krishna Consciousness (ISKCON)

might be described as a Hindu Vaisneva sect that was imported
from India to the United States in 1964. The late founder of this
missionary movement was A.C. Bhaktivedanta Swami Prabhu-
pada who arrived in New York off the boat from India, sat down
under a tree in Tompkins Park, and began chanting the name of
Krishna. He attracted the attention of young hippies disillusioned
with the drug scene, and within five years he had established
ISKCON temples all over the world.

In this highly visible religious minority members adopt eastern
clothing and the men shave their heads – and they are intensely
evangelical. They reject North American culture and worldly at-
tachments which are regarded as *maya*, or illusion, and are dedicated to living the traditional Vedic way of life and surrendering
to Krishna, the Supreme Personality of the Godhead. They also
espouse a radical body-spirit dualism in which they emphasize the
transient nature of material life and the need to prepare for the
reincarnation cycle. The aim of the spirit-soul is to advance up the
scale of purity until, no longer subject to the laws of *karma* or cause
and effect, she (the soul is female in relation to her Lord) can
become one with Krishna and dwell eternally in *Vrindavana*, depicted as a beautiful heavenly garden.

Upon initiation, members must recite before the guru the four
vows: the promise to refrain from meat-eating, non-procreative
sex, drugs, and gambling. In addition, they must promise to recite
the Hare Krishna *mahamantra* (great mantra) daily, which they
believe purifies the soul and expresses their love for God.

Given their commitment to an ascetic life and their radical separation from the world, it is not surprising that in ISKCON literature
AIDS is associated with the pursuit of sensual gratification, with
the laws of *karma*, and with the inevitable decay and illusory nature
of the physical body. There is, however, surprisingly little mention
of the disease in their magazine, *Back to Godhead*. This might be
accounted for by the institutionalization of charisma since the
death of their founder in 1977, and by ISKCON's rejection of Western
culture and conscious reconstruction of ancient Vedic society –
resulting in a lack of interest concerning current social problems.

One moral lesson derived from AIDS is a reminder of the ephemeral nature of the body and the eternal nature of the spirit-soul which inhabits it. Basanudas Prabhu makes this point in the *Bombay Newsletter* (1990):

> Why should we continue to suffer, chasing transient enjoyment in a contaminated world, when we can have eternal, unlimited enjoyment in the spiritual world with Krsna? . . . AIDS is bad, but the disease of birth in the material world is always fatal!

Srila Bhakti Abhay Charan Swami (1990) of the Brooklyn temple also finds in AIDS an occasion to preach a radical body/soul dichotomy:

> We are suffering because of being identified with the body which has to get sick, old and die. But in the Vedic literature it is explained that we are not these bodies. Our real identity is spirit soul. And anything that may occur to these bodies does not affect our soul in any way.

Mother Yadurani Devi Dasi of the Brooklyn temple argues that the pursuit of sexual pleasure perpetuates that illusion, and condemns scientists for dispensing material knowledge as opposed to the spiritual knowledge taught in the *Vedas*:[6]

> Materialistic so-called authorities recommend various insipid remedies, such as banning prostitutes from having sex with foreigners, making prostitutes raise their prices, distributing free condoms, etc. None of these concocted solutions will work, because the real cause of AIDS is not a virus – it is the sinful habit of illicit sex. The disease is just the inevitable karmic reaction. But none of the 'great scientists' can think to ban illicit sex!

She contrasts ISKCON standards of sexual self-control with the larger society's permissive attitudes towards 'illicit sex':

> Sexually transmitted diseases . . . could easily be stopped if people would only give up illicit sex. It is recommended in all scriptures . . .

that one should have sex only to procreate children in his lawfully wedded wife. And even then there are restrictions and regulations to be followed for first-class progeny. The would-be parents chant fifty rounds of the Hare Krsna mantra – *Hare Krishna Hare Krishna, Krishna Krishna Hare Hare, Hare Rama Hare Rama, Rama Rama Hare Hare* – before conceiving. They only make this attempt once in a month, a few days after the menstrual cycle.

Srila Bhakti Abhay Charan Swami (1990) sees in the advent of AIDS a lesson in the laws of *karma*:

The arrival of AIDS in our society makes us reflect with urgency about the responsibility of every single one of our actions. Everyone who has AIDS is like someone who is drowning slowly and painfully without being able to receive help . . . This is simply another defeat that all of humanity is experiencing due to the ignorance of the laws of cause and effect.

He suggests PWAs are receiving karmic reactions from misdeeds in previous lifetimes. For this god-brother, the message of AIDS is, 'Wake up and realize your spiritual identity!'

The law of *karma*, like any other universal law, works impartially, providing exactly what we deserve . . . The disease generally appears as a reaction for some committed mistake. In this case, the mistake consists mainly in maintaining a bodily concept of life . . . For this reason, the worst that can occur to a person with AIDS is not the disease itself – but to die in ignorance of the real cause of such a disease. He cannot rectify his behavior without the proper knowledge of who he is and what is his or her constitutional position: service to the Supreme Personality of the Godhead. Without this knowledge, a person is doomed to continue this same suffering in the next life after death.

The presence of the HIV virus in semen resonates with traditional Vedic medicine, which holds that the loss of semen in sexual indulgence results in weakness and premature death:

The great sage Narada Muni was a *naisthika-brahmacari* – that is, he never had a sex life. He was consequently an ever-green youth . . . It requires great strength to resist a woman's attraction . . . Those who are too much sexually addicted become victims of *Jara* and very soon their life-span is shortened. Without utilizing the human form of life for Krsna consciousness, the victims of *Jara* die very soon in this world. (*Srimad Bhagavatam* 4.27.21)

(An ISKCON leader's comment on this passage was, 'We can see here how AIDS was foretold in the scriptures of 5000 years ago!')

In searching for references in ancient Sanskrit texts offering guidelines on how to approach the contemporary phenomenon of homosexuals with AIDS from a traditional Vedic perspective, ISKCON leaders pointed to a passage denouncing an esoteric sect of *saddhus* (holy man) who engaged in homosexual acts as part of their spiritual practice. Ironically, these misguided 'rascals' will be reborn on a higher scale of purity than the devoted husband, who will return as a woman. Although homosexual *saddhus* will be punished by being reborn as 'dogs, hogs and monkeys' (actually *lower* on the purity scale than a woman), even these base forms of life will be spiritually elevated upon death simply by living in the holy city of Vrndavana:

The city called Gramaka, which is approached through the lower gate of Asuri [the genitals] is meant for sex, which is very pleasing to common men who are simply fools and rascals . . . When the world becomes degraded . . . the rectum and the genitalia are taken very seriously as the centers of all activity. Even in such a sacred place as Vrndavana, India, unintelligent men pass off this rectal and genital business as spiritual activity. Such people are called *sahajiya*. According to their philosophy, through sexual indulgence one can elevate oneself to the spiritual platform . . . To rectify these rascals and fools is very difficult . . . For this reason, Vrndavana is no longer visited by intelligent men.

It can be concluded that Vrndavana has become degenerate due to these *sahajiyas*, yet from the spiritual point of view, Vrndavana is the only place where all these sinful persons can be rectified by means of taking birth in the forms of dogs, hogs, and monkeys. By living in Vrndavana as a dog, hog, or monkey, the living entity can be elevated to the spiritual platform in the next life. (*Srimad Bhaga-vatam* 4.29.14)

How this esoteric knowledge might be of use to modern gays was not explained. It would appear that ISKCON leaders, in consulting ancient Vedic scriptures for clues to understanding this modern disease, find that AIDS is not necessarily any more significant than other bodily infirmity. It is just another reminder that the body and spirit are utterly separate, and that the pursuit of sense gratification will affect one's *karma* adversely. ISKCON espouses a cyclic view of time and is not a millenarian movement. AIDS, for Krishna devotees, is just another building block in the wall surrounding their sect – a symbol of the corruption and illusory nature of western 'civilization.'

The Messianic Communities

The Messianic Communities, also known as the Northeast Kingdom Community Church, was originally founded by Eugene Elbert Spriggs (known as Yoneq) in Chattanooga, Tennessee, in 1972. Emerging from the Jesus People Revival in the mid-1970s, the Community looks toward the return of Jesus or 'Yahshua' whom they believe will claim His 'Pure and Spotless Bride' – or His own people, obedient to his word. Members buy and renovate old houses to set up communal households. A high value is placed on 'raising up a people' through marriages based on 'the rock of fidelity' and training children in the 'way they should go.' Members adopt Hebrew names, and the women wear headscarves when publicly praying or prophesying to denote their submission to God's created order. Their husbands, in turn, are 'covered' by Yahshua. The Communities hold public gatherings on the Shabbat of Friday to Saturday that combine the old-fashioned revival meeting with the barn dance. Men and women prophesy and offer testimonies of faith and thanksgiving. Parents and children dance and sing songs composed by their own people, accompanied by hand-made Celtic and Appalachian instruments (Palmer, 1994). The original Community in Island Pond, Vermont, has spread through New England, Manitoba, Brazil, France, and New Zealand. The group is evangelical and currently numbers around 1,500 members.[7]

The Messianic Communities welcome outsiders to their gatherings and offer visitors one night's accommodation with a meal and board, which this researcher and her children accepted on several occasions. One morning, while helping in the kitchen, I observed that outsiders' dishes were dipped in bleach. In response to my question on AIDS precautions, an elder informed me that aspiring members with past histories of drug abuse or sexual promiscuity are asked to undergo AIDS tests, and that the Community has its own blood bank.

The Messianic Community's position on AIDS falls into the judgmental category, reflecting their roots in the Jesus Movement. They explicitly state that the plague is the result of individuals' going against God's will and is a clear sign that heterosexual monogamy with procreative intent within the covenant of marriage is the only form of sexual expression acceptable to God.

The Community's *Freepaper* came out with a statement on homosexuality and AIDS in a 1992 article called 'Back to the Garden: Death of a Snake Charmer.' A member mourns the death of a gay friend, praising his talents and charm, but condemning his orientation:

> Bob played with snakes, ate with snakes, and even slept with snakes. In order to receive the first embrace of his male lover, Bob had to stifle his screaming conscience ... Bob's life *was* a tragic waste, not because he was afflicted with AIDS but because he suppressed his instinctive knowledge of what is good and true, trading his dignity for pleasure ... Yet when Bob was injected with the final lethal venom of AIDS, his degenerate society mourned the passing of a hero. ('Back to the Garden,' 1992:34)

The authority of Leviticus is invoked: 'If there is a man who lies with a male as those who lie with a woman, both of them have committed a detestable act; they shall surely be put to death.' This introduces the article 'Homosexuals,' which launches an uncompromising condemnation of homosexuality: 'SO HOMOSEXUALS ARE BRINGING THE EARTH CLOSER AND CLOSER TO DEVASTATION, and the wrath of God will come upon the whole earth because Man tolerates what is disgusting to him.'

AIDS is clearly considered a graphic example of the consequences of sin and anarchy, which the Messianic Communities perceive as rife in the larger society, and is used to draw the line that divides God's People from the sinners who are doomed to everlasting death. AIDS defines the boundaries between the two societies: Yahshua's church and the wasteland surrounding it.

The lecture, 'AIDS: A Looming Shadow,' was delivered by Charash, a teacher, and Yonah, an elder, at the *Religion and AIDS* seminar organized and chaired by myself and Professor Arvind Sharma at McGill University, on 1 December 1990. (Permission to quote from their speech was granted by Charash, on the condition that the address of their community would be included.)

These members interpret AIDS as a judgment on sinful humanity and a sign of the fearful recompense 'justly due' to those who violate God's natural laws and ignore His commandments:

> We look at AIDS from what I guess you'd call the apocalyptic point of view ... we see that AIDS is a judgment on humanity ... for its flagrant denial of God's word. It's a forerunner of the pestilences included in the Book of Revelation, and also in the Gospels, Luke 21. Man is opening up the floodgates of sin by tolerating what is obviously reprehensible!

The Old Testament laws concerning the use of blood, food, and sexuality as divinely ordained are underlined:

> We see that this natural sense of what human beings ought to do and shouldn't do, that touches upon sexual practices, that touches on what we should do with blood, how we keep clean – the thousands of things it touches! – these things have been superseded by a higher wisdom of our modern Western society. There is no

longer a proper fear of consequences at the root of our actions, we can just about move around and do whatever we please. This has been made possible by a lifting of custom, tradition, and taboo everywhere. All over the Earth people are free to do whatever they want, and this makes possible sin on the grandest scale imaginable.

The universal scale and apocalyptic message of the cataclysm is emphasized:

What is to be done? We don't see AIDS as just threatening the particular individuals that practise sin. It doesn't just threaten the homosexual, the bisexual, the drug abuser, or just the sexually immoral. The implications touch the entire human race ... It's not as if the human race deserves to escape the coming wrath! We don't see that it is worthy to be saved, for God to hold back His wrath. We as a community do take steps of hygiene regarding the casual passing of AIDS. But we see that beyond everything, we human beings must remember our Creator and find our way back to His laws and His standards – obviously, I'm painting a pretty grim picture here.

Finally, the role of the Messianic Communities during this unprecedented crisis was outlined:

The only reason the God of Heaven will hold this terrible force of destruction back, is so that He can have time to raise up a people. AIDS is only the first in a series of judgments that will culminate in the return of the Son of Man. We call Him Yahshua. These plagues, pestilences, wars, rumours of wars, all manner of things you read about in the Book of Revelation, are pointing out to us that we, as human beings, are departing from the Divine Plane. The outcome of this process will be two distinct societies: a society that is materially rich but absolutely devoid of any contact with its Creator. This spiritually bankrupt society will be characterized by drug and alcohol abuse and illicit sexual practices with resulting plagues and diseases. And there will be another society, raised up alongside it, that will be characterized by obeying the truth of the Creator, and by a life of unity, of caring about one other, and there will be wholeness, there will restoration in its midst. (Charash [Bill Smith] and Yonah [David Jones], The Community in Island Pond, Box 443, Island Pond, Vermont 05846)

The Children of God/The Family

The Family is a Christian millenarian, communal missionary movement. Its founder David Berg, his wife Jane, and their four teenagers were conspicuously successful in their missionary efforts among the 'lost generation' of hippies on Huntingdon Beach, California, in 1968, and the Children of God was born. The movement has had a high turnover rate, for around 36,000 members have defected. In recent years, the second generation, who outnumber the adults two to one, have been encouraged to assume positions of responsibility within the group's hierarchy.[8]

The Family are Christian fundamentalist whose beliefs are firmly based on the Bible, but they also emphasize the *Mo Letters* of David Berg, the 'Lord's Endtime Prophet.' They left America in the early 1970s in the expectation that the comet Kahoutek would destroy America, but have recently returned home for a final harvest of souls who must 'get saved' in preparation for Jesus' return. They expect to play a key role in the cosmic battle against the forces of Satan, after which the Golden Pyramid will descend from Heaven to inaugurate the millennium.

Berg's minor theological innovations and communications with the spirit world have antagonized mainstream Christian churches. Some parents whose children have 'forsaken all for Jesus' have joined forces with the handful of embittered defectors and the anticult movement to accuse the Children of God of 'brainwashing' their sudden converts. But the weight of public criticism has focused on The Family's sexual practices.

The Family's sexual ethics are based on the 'Law of Love,' as expounded by David Berg. The Law of Love draws on biblical passages to outlaw incest, birth control, abortion, and sodomy, but presents a positive attitude towards sex and the body, summed up in the *Mo Letters* as 'Revolutionary Sex.' Revolutionary Sex rebelled against the Christian church's 'prohibitory and condemnatory attitude towards sex' and encouraged sexual sharing outside marriage between consenting heterosexual adults, and permits masturbation and nudity as God-given needs (Melton, 1995).

While this development simply 'Christianized' the hippie generation's sexual revolution, a more radical step was taken when Berg and his young consort, Maria, pioneered the 'Flirty Fishing Ministry' in the mid-1970s. This involved using sexual attractiveness and sexual favours to win souls for Jesus, to bring new members in, and (incidentally) to drum up financial support for the movement. Between 1977 and 1987, their official statistics claimed over 100,000 people had been personally led to Jesus Christ as a direct result of the Flirty Fishing ('FFing') Ministry. This unusual outreach method has invited accusations of immorality from other Christians, along with charges of operating prostitution rings. Anticultists have attacked The Family in pamphlets such as the one produced by the No Longer Children Support Group based in Richmond, British Columbia:

> 'The Family'/Children of God/Family of Love/Music with Meaning/Heaven's Magic – An Urgent Warning!
> Soon scores of COG members became outright prostitutes, leading to hundreds becoming infected with sexually transmitted diseases such as herpes (which reached near-epidemic proportions in some areas).

Family members, however, insist that 'Ffing' was consistent with a 'sacrificial ministry' and that its 'fruit was good' when performed in their understanding of the true spirit of Christian love.

As the Children of God matured through The Family of Love phase and into The Family, they have gradually become more conservative, and the threat of AIDS has played a significant role in this transformation. In a Mo Letter in March 1983, the leadership expressed concern about reports of sexually transmitted diseases passing between homes. This letter, entitled 'Ban the Bomb,' prohibited sexual sharing *between* homes, while allowing it to continue *within* individual communal homes. In 1984 the letter 'No Sex for Babes' laid down the rule that new members must remain celibate for the first six months in the home. Disobedience to this rule became an excommunicable offence in 1989.

In 1987 the leadership expressed a strong concern that AIDS might invade their close-knit commune through Flirty Fishing. A letter came out in the October 1987 edition of the *Good News!* magazine (GN 287) called 'Special AIDS Edition!' Instructions noted, 'Can be read to close friends and long-time fish if necessary!':

> Several reports have come in about potential new disciples desiring to come into the Family who turned out to be carriers of . . . AIDS. To help protect our worldwide Family from the 'plague of the Egyptians' . . . all new disciples must be medically *tested* before joining the Family, then tested again six months later before they are cleared to share sexually with other family members.

The rule that 'Babes' abstain from sex for first six months 'so they don't get all entangled in a romantic affair that could hinder their spiritual growth' was more urgently enforced because of the 'scourge of AIDS.'

David Berg's comment on the possibility of faith healing was, 'The Lord can heal anything, even AIDS, but it's better to build a fence at the top of the hill than a hospital at the bottom.'

New Flirty Fishing guidelines were laid down in the letter called, 'The New Sexless FFing or Condom Revolution':

> It would be absolutely tragic if The Family were to unwisely allow this horrible affliction to enter in and spread. Because of its long gestation period it could, no doubt – except for God's protection and mercy – spread quite rapidly through our ranks, due to our sexual liberties in sharing. I'm not trying to be any kind of doom-sayer or . . . freaked out . . . but we've already seen . . . other sexually transmitted diseases, which thank the Lord He has healed and delivered us from. But the hitch with AIDS is that it *doesn't* clear up, except of course by an absolute, total miracle of God . . . It just seems like our FFers are putting themselves at risk . . . caution them to be extra prayerful and careful about who they go to bed with (and be sure they wear *condoms*!).

This new policy had emotional ramifications. The letter 'Condom Battles and Victories!' announces, 'girls report many of their long-time fish are hurt at being distanced, excluded from The Family by having to wear a condom.' But David Berg's tough response was, 'I think this is going to cure a lot of the promiscuity and profligacy and wild circulation of some of our FFers . . . concentrating more on *money* than they were on catching fish and making solid converts and disciples.'

AIDS provides an opportunity for the Lord's Endtime Prophet to censure homosexuality and conjure up visions of God's wrath:

> I tell you, the people who don't keep the rules will pay! Just like the sodomites are paying now! See, the Lord is not going to let them find a cure! Those who deserve it, are going to get their punishment whether they like it or not. I think this is the beginning of the final judgments, final curses, final plagues!

What is interesting, for our purposes, is the fact that, in spite of The Family's notoriety for free love and Flirty Fishing, only two of their commune members have, to my knowledge, actually died of AIDS – and that was in the mid-1980s. Their authority structure is strong, and the rules were strictly enforced. Prophylactic measures including quarantine, testing, and the segregation of potentially infected new disciples were sufficient to protect the small, self-contained communal homes. Today The Family bans sex with outsiders, homosexuality and sex with minors – on pain of excommunication – but continues to encourage heterosexual 'sharing' between consenting adults, true to the principles of sexual communism and mystical eroticism expressed in the *Mo Letters* of their founder.

The Politics of Isolation

Metaphorical thinking has not inhibited these groups from paying attention to scientific reports or adopting rational prophylactic actions. Unimpeded by their religious rhetoric, these communities have investigated the available medical literature and quickly instituted effective precautions to safeguard their members. It is interesting to note that even the two free-love communities, the Raelians and The Family, appear to be 'AIDS-free zones' today.

Leaders in these communal movements have all been faced with the situation in which a person with AIDS has shown up at their gatherings, seeking spiritual solace or wishing to join the community. They have been forced to hammer out hasty policies, since it is a far more threatening situation to live communally with a contagious person than to share a pew with one on Sunday. While it might be against their philosophy to reject those in need, there is a strong imperative to protect the community. The Messianic Communities demand tests from aspiring members who have a 'sinful' history before they can be baptized into the 'Body.' Unificationists must undergo HIV tests before getting married in the Blessing. I am acquainted with at least two other new religious communes who also employ mandatory AIDS testing. The Sullivanians, a therapeutic commune in New York, undergo tests for HIV every three months.[9] The Free Daist Communion tests its members before they can visit their spiritual master, Love Da Ananda, on his island in Fiji.[10] In every case, the threat of AIDS is referred to by group leaders to reinforce the particular sexual program of the community, whether it is free love with condoms in the Rajneesh Movement, celibacy in ISKCON, or arranged marriages in the Unification Church.

Our postmillennialist groups each have a model of the 'Perfect Man' who is on a higher scale of purity than the rest of humanity. This quest for the pure involves a rather obsessive preoccupation with bodily fluids. Jehovah's Witnesses and Unificationists hold strong convictions on blood, its consumption, and contamination. The Rajneeshee, described in Chapter 4, regard *all* excretions, even sweat and tears, as potentially contaminating. Underlying this treatment of the body as an impermeable vessel is the idea that by blocking the orifices connecting the individual to the material world, one can force open new and hidden channels to the spiritual realm. Unificationists who are 'restored' begin to open their five 'spiritual senses' and see into the spirit world; Rajneeshee hold their breath and hyperventilate in past lives workshops to experience flashes of previous incarnations. The Raelians (see Chapter 4) stimulate their senses as a means of telepathic communication with the Elohim.

In all these groups their spiritual strategies for coping with AIDS are consistent with their body symbols and millenarian expectations. For Rajneesh and Rael, it is scientists who will be the midwives in the birth of the millennium. Therefore they recommend condoms, which serve a similar function to a liturgical vestment among their followers. Wearing a condom reinforces the autonomy of the New Man, godlike and impermeable in his detachment from the past and from family ties. The humble condom is an element in the ritual, for through sexual discipline initiates strive for an experiential transcendance of death through an expanded awareness in the present.

The notion that the loss of semen resulted in 'feeblemindedness' or senility was promoted by nineteenth-century physicians and discussed in the writings of Sylvester Graham and Thomas Low Nichols (Kern, 1981:375). Almost parodying this fear, we find the Oneida Perfectionists, a nineteenth-century commune in southern New York, practising free love, but avoiding procreation through *coitus reservati*. As postmillennialists they believed they could enjoy extraordinary longevity and perfect health so long as they avoided the sin of 'selfish love' and retained their semen. Unconsciously echoing their forebears in free love, the Rajneesh and Raelians reject monogamy and procreation and use sex as a path to the divine and as a means to create an elite super race. Thus, their use of the condom could be seen as a modern version of the Victorian obsession with 'spermatic economics,' and their preoccupation with AIDS might be just another postmillennialist attempt to find 'sexual solutions to death.'

FOUR

Spiritual Politics and Sadhanas

Kashi Ashram, The Raelian Movement, The Church Universal and Triumphant, Ramtha, The Vajradhatu Buddhist International Church

The members of these new religious movements do not live in communes – with the exception of their core group workers, who live in the intense, emotional circle of *communitas* surrounding the charismatic leader (Weber, 1968), devoting their lives to the goals of the movement. The main body of disciples of Kashi, the Church Universal, and Vajradhatu live in society and are encouraged to pursue the worldly goals of health, wealth, and personal happiness. Disciples sign up for periodic spiritual retreats at these Shaivite, Theosophical, or Buddhist ashrams where they receive meditation instruction, inspiration, and guidance along their spiritual path or *sadhana*. Apprentices of Ramtha and Rael enrol in occasional workshops where they are trained in magical/therapeutic techniques enabling them to tap into hidden forces or entities useful for personal and secular ends. Consistent with these relaxed boundaries, the AIDS threat is not seen as an occasion to exert greater social control. While it is still a 'spiritual disease,' it is not endowed with the same cosmic significance found in the speeches of Rajneesh and Reverend Moon.

Kashi Ashram

The Kashi ashram is an interfaith religious community in Florida, based primarily on the Shaivite tradition. The River Fund, established in 1990, is the service arm of the ashram, and is explained in brochures as 'a non-profit volunteer-based service organization dedicated to serving the needs of those affected by HIV and AIDS and other life-threatening diseases.' Kashi has become a thriving pilgrimage centre and respite for PWAs and their loved ones. The Memorial Boardwalk was built in 1991 beside the Sebastian River, a spot secluded by tall palms and oak trees where friends and family of those with AIDS who have passed on can sit on benches bearing their names. There is also a pond where ashes of the cremated are scattered.

Ma Jaya Sati Bhagavati, a Jewish woman in her fifties, is the ashram's founder, and a shaman/guru of the art of dying. She was born Joyce Green, from the 'holy land of Brooklyn,' and is famous for her street-wise *chutzpah* and total commitment to people with AIDS. Her ashram has been described as a 'Lourdes for gays' where she presides, equipped with 'enough piercings and bangles to set off an alarm at LAX' (Monnette, n.d.). She receives her students and visitors in traditional guru style, but she is also a warm-hearted Jewish Mama who hugs the old, young, sick, infectious, and well, and teaches others to hug. She flaunts her street lingo, 'shrieking in Brooklynese' and 'braying with excitement,' and shocks her listeners with vulgar jokes. National Books Award winner Paul Monnette describes the red *tilak* on her forehead as 'Revlon bright' and notes she was swathed in 'more veils than Salome, but none to cover her beaming face.' Her charisma is mitigated by self-satire: 'There can only be one Holy Mother around here, and I am it, so why don't you all just shut up!'

In 1976 Ma Jaya set up an interfaith ashram in Roseland, Florida, called Kashi ('city of light'), and proceeded to care for unwanted and abused children. As they grew up, she started a school. Today the school has a good reputation and is attended by outside children. Around a hundred disciples or *chelas* live in permanent residence, and the ashram attracts a constant stream of pilgrims and visitors. Ma insists that residents should remain vegetarian and celibate and celibacy seems good sense in a place where so many victims of the new plague are congregated.

Ma Jaya Sati Bhagavati fills a gaping *lacuna* on the American scene; she offers those afflicted with HIV a ritual approach to dying and an adequate and comforting philosophy of death. Her first lesson in death came in 1950, when her own mother was in a cancer ward, having had one breast and a lung removed when Joyce was ten years old. When Joyce asked *why* God allowed this to happen to good people, her mother replied, 'Don't ever ask why because you will never get an answer. Just pray for what you want in life and God in his wisdom will figure out what you need. Always remember to thank God for what you already have.' Later, on seeing her daughter pray, she said, 'Honey, don't look up for God to hear you. Close your eyes and look into your heart.' Joyce writes, 'in that crowded ward – which reminded you of the depths of Hell – I found God. Inside of me.'

Ma's declared mission is to make herself available to people who need to learn how to die: As she once explained:

> Months before the physical death, the person has asked me to teach them how to die. And we've danced; we've danced with a little bit of life, and the dance has been so profound, so deep – a never-ending waltz because I, their Ma, have taught them detachment.

She claims that at age thirty-two, as a Jewish wife and overweight mother of three children, suddenly Christ appeared to her. She was studying yoga as a means to lose weight and practising breathing exercises at the foot of the stairs when Christ appeared. Ma received stigmata on her hands and feet in imitation of Christ, and every Good Friday develops red welts on her hands. Like the shaman who astral-travels between the world of the living and the spirits of the afterworld so as to facilitate the journey of the dying, Ma has beheld Kali, the goddess of death, and engaged in long conversations with her on the meaning of the 'extreme amount of pain at the end of the horrendous disease, AIDS' (*River Fund* newsletter, 1994:29). She credits Kali for giving her lessons on detachment, forgiveness, and *karma*.

> I, the Mother, have seen now in this time of the AIDS virus that the true seeker of knowledge learns in the shortest time space known to man or God . . . I have seen the suffering suffer enough for a million lifetimes as they fight this terrible disease, AIDS.

Sometimes Ma Jaya appears to embody the goddess Kali in her writing:

> So I walk and talk and run and hold and scream and yell and carry on and teach them all that death does have a heart, that they need to go into the center of their own heart to find death's heart . . . where AIDS has no hand, where cancer has no claws. I am called the Mother and I, the Mother, hold my children close to my breast so they can feel the fullness of life. When they die a piece of me dies. But I drink as I pour and get ready for the next person who asks 'Ma, teach me how to die.'

Ma is scornful of Christian sanctimony, and is a harsh critic of priests and ministers who discriminate against gays and transvestites:

> One cold morning as I was working at the County Home in West Palm Beach, I heard a minister screaming at a young man . . . telling him that his AIDS was a retribution from God . . . I threw the minister out and jumped in bed with this young man, holding him tight.

Ma Jaya visits patients in county homes and hospitals and kisses them in spite of their lesions. She told Cardinal O'Connor that Christ would never have refused a dying man in drag (*Shambala Sun*, March 1995). She rejects the notion of a judgmental, punitive deity:

> Do not judge God. I'm sure God did not orchestrate the holocaust or the cancer that took my mothe's life when I was 13. I'm sure God didn't say 'let there be AIDS.' I'm also just as sure that God gave us the will and the way to fight all the above).' (*River Fund* newsletter, n.d.)

Gays love her, for she acknowledges the creativity, vitality, and pathos of their alternative world. An obituary to Agni, a frequent visitor to the ashram ('often dressed in his favorite leather outfit, chains choker and all'), notes that his parting gift to Ma was a performance of his drag show: 'A large crowd of us filled the bar to overflowing on that rainy night. With dress and heels replacing leather, it was a great send-off show. Underneath the unique, always outrageous outfits, Agni was gentle . . . and even quiet. Many people didn't know that one of his favorite hobbies was crocheting afghans' *(River Fund* newsletter, Fall, 1994).

The late Paul Monnette observed that many of Ma Jaya's followers have already sampled other spiritual solutions, and are disillusioned by the New Age gurus with upbeat messages and expensive panaceas for PWAs. He contrasts Ma's good-samaritan approach and acceptance of the dying to the systems in which the 'dying were losers' (as in the *Course in Miracles*) that tell you 'anger will kill you faster than AIDS.' He exposes the hidden cruelty in the 'various denial systems purveyed by Marianne [Williamson] and Louise [Hay] – New Age ladies that drew the line at visiting the dying [and who] make people feel that if they *do* get sicker they weren't loving their lesions enough or keeping up with their positive imaging.'

Ma performs weddings for gay, lesbian, and straight couples: 'Having married man to man and woman to woman, I find that gay marriages are just as filled with love – and sometimes with greater love – as most straight marriages.' She also cooks spicy tomato sauce for Project Angelfood, a volunteer organization that provides meals-on-wheels for PWAs at home.[11]

Ma Jaya says, 'There is only one religion and it is called kindness.'

The Raelian Movement

The Raelian movement was founded by a Frenchman, Claude Vorilhon (Rael to his followers), in 1973, as the result of his alleged encounter with space aliens who entrusted him with a message. This message concerns the origins of human life: these extraterrestrials, called 'Elohim,' created us from their own DNA in their laboratories and 'implanted' us on earth. Rael's mission, as the last of forty prophets (cross-bred between Elohim and mortal women), is to warn humankind that since 1945 and Hiroshima, we have entered the 'Age of the Apocalypse' in which we have the choice of destroying ourselves with nuclear weapons, or making the leap into planetary consciousness as inheritors of the scientific knowledge of our creators. This will enable our species in the future to clone ourselves in *our* 'own image' and to populate other planets.

The movement in 1996 claims around 35,000 members worldwide, distributed mainly throughout France, Quebec, Japan, and several African countries, and hopes through Rael's books and lectures to unite all religions in a de-mythologized interpretation of scripture as the true history of the Elohim's space colonization program. Denying the existence of God or the soul, Rael presents as the only hope of immortality a regeneration through science by means of process similar to cloning. To this end, new members must undergo a 'baptism' during which, Raelians believe, the Elohim hover close to earth and register the initiates' DNA codes on their ships' computers.[12]

The Raelians have a strong millenarian focus and await the descent of the Elohim and the forty prophets in spaceships in Jerusalem where they intend to build an intergalactic embassy sometime before 2025. Meanwhile, Rael advises Raelians not to marry or exacerbate the planetary overpopulation problem, but to commune with the wonder of the universe by exploring their sexuality. Raelians can participate during the summer in a one-week workshop held on a campsite where nudity is permitted, where they practise 'sensual meditation,' a technique of awakening the mind through awakening the body.

Rael's statement on AIDS appears in the group's magazine, *Apocalypse* (May, June, and July 1988), and is entitled: 'Vivre, c'est risquer!' True to his mission to demystify religion, Rael begins by deploring the opportunistic moralizings of the established churches over the AIDS problem: 'l'apparition du SIDA qui leur permet de vanter les mérites de la chastité, la monogamie, de l'hétérosexualité, la fidelité.' He equates the notion of divine punishment with the 'primitif' response to the bubonic plague and syphilis in European history, and comments, 'Quelle stupidité!' For him, the situation calls for an intelligent, scientific approach to the danger, in the footsteps of 'nos ancêtres' the Elohim, who have weathered epidemics on other planets; first, by avoiding stress which weakens the body's defences ('c'est scientifiquement re-connu') and next, by maintaining a healthy diet (coffee, tea, sugar, and tobacco are mentioned as not indigenous to Europe, therefore unknown to our ancestors). These substances, as well as alcohol, are proscribed for members in the Raelian hierarchy. Finally, he affirms that only the most intelligent will survive, since 'les imbéciles' will rely on God and prayer for protection. Rael made the use of the condom obligatory for members in 1976, and he notes that by anticipating the current promotion of 'cette petite merveille de la science' his people have shown themselves to be 'les plus conscients.'

Alternative means of transmission are not to be worried about since we can't live in a sterile universe and 'vivre, c'est risquer!' Indeed, by accepting risk we can enrich and strengthen ourselves, Rael insists.

Rael concludes his message on AIDS with a rather explicit testimonial to 'la poésie' of the sexual act and reassures his followers that the use of the condom should not detract from their ability to 'lever la conscience' and experience 'tout l'amour du monde' and 'toute la sensualité de l'univers.'

The Raelian Movement in Quebec is one of the most compassionate of all the new religions in Canada, and offers the most practical assistance to PWAs (known as sidéens' in Quebec). This is mainly due to the efforts of Marie-Marcelle Godbout, 'Priest-Guide,' who works for SIDA Montréal as a counsellor and specializes in women with AIDS. Although she makes a point of not pushing the message on her clients, she feels that the positive values and insights into humanity she has gained from her experience in the movement are of benefit in her counselling work. At the last tri-annual meeting of the Raelian Movement on 13 December 1990 at the Holiday Inn in Longueil, Godbout had invited a PWA to speak, but unfortunately he was too weak to attend, so instead she conducted a meditation session in which the assembled members sent out healing vibrations to the him.

Victor LeGendre, the former National Guide of Canada, made a statement outlining the Raelian Movement's formal response to the AIDS crisis for the *Religion and Aids* conference held in Montreal on 1 December 1990. In this response, the Raelians seize the opportunity to declare their atheism and their faith in science. They reject the notion of sin and the 'wrath-of-God thesis,' and affirm the physicist's mystical vision of the unity of all life:

> AIDS, according to Raelian philosophy, is not a God-sent disease to punish man for his evil doings. Since we deny the existence of God, we are atheists. AIDS, as any other plague on this planet, is a challenge to be overcome. By the grace of science this illness will be cured. Human beings must elevate their consciousness to become more sensitive to the problem . . . whatever afflicts one individual touches the rest of humanity. The individual and humanity are indivisible and in relationship.

He affirms the moral worth of PWAs and the Raelian commitment to sensual pleasure and sexual freedom:

> A person with HIV is just as dignified and worthy a person as a person without this disease. A venereal disease is not a shameful disease. All sexual or sensual pleasure is good for a person's balance as long as he or she expresses their sexuality in a conscious way. Consequently, our society must provide moral support to a person infected with AIDS.

He outlines the precautionary measures adopted by the movement and the use of creative visualization and fasting to heal HIV-positive Raelians:

> During the seminar that Rael gives over the summer, we teach the importance of a balanced sexual life. We emphasize the importance of using the condom, which we have been distributing at our seminars for fourteen years. We educate our members in the dangers of STD, and in some cases, fasting was used as a means of purifying oneself of the virus. We have a member in France . . . and he's taken two cases of HIV and . . . undergone a long fast – 30 or 40 days. They underwent creative visualization and meditated – and they got rid

of it. We don't have enough cases to present it formally, but at least two people have been cured.

In contrast to the isolating response of communal movements, the Raelians adopt an activist approach towards AIDS as well as towards other social issues. Raelians stage public demonstrations and court the media during their Planetary Week in April, in an attempt to influence public opinion towards 'racial, sexual and religious minorities.' Rael advises his followers, 'We must not *break* the law, but that does not mean we cannot seek to *change* the law!' Perhaps because of their world-affirming, non-sectarian orientation, they do not see the virus as particularly catching and propose pragmatic solutions to the AIDS crisis:

> Society must work on a plan of prevention so as to halt the virus spreading further [and] support scientific research so as to find a quick solution to this problem. We must use science to remedy and compensate for the wrongs of humanity.

In their concern for the well-being of PWAs, they fit the compassionate response:

> As far as the affective aspect is concerned, any negativity towards HIV people must be abolished. The guides in our movement are doing everything they can to facilitate the adjustment of affected persons, and must exert themselves to change this primitive perception of AIDS victims. We must strive to elevate the collective consciousness so that each human has a place in our collectivity . . . therefore society must allow each HIV person to live a decent life.

The Raelians don't discourage PWAs from attending their meetings. One PWA filled in a questionnaire that my students were distributing at the 13 December 1994 'Transmission of the Cellular Plan.' Every summer at the Sensual Meditation Camp the guides remind the campers to scrub the shower stalls with bleach after use and to use condoms if they are with a new partner during the sexual experiments that are encouraged in the seminar.

Since Raelians regard the extraterrestrial scientists who created life on planet Earth as older brothers rather than as *dei ex machina*, they advocate human self-reliance rather than prayer for divine intervention:

> The Elohim do not intervene directly to help men sort out their problems. They consider us as capable of overcoming our own problems with our wisdom and consciousness. They . . . recognize the intelligence of the humans they have created . . . because they are his creators. Out of love and respect for the human species, they prefer to let men decide for themselves. The destiny of homo sapiens is in our hands, not in the hands of those who created us. It is up to us to gain or lose our lives on this planet.

On the cosmological level, AIDS is a reminder of the universe's vast infinity, which speaks of humanity's insignificance in relation to space, and yet, within the framework of human consciousness, speaks of the profound importance of our survival as a species:

> Infinity is composed of space and time . . . In Raelian theory, infinity is not conscious of itself. Only the human being can be conscious of himself, of his humanity, and of his universe. Therefore, as infinity lacks consciousness or a distinct identity, AIDS does not represent a problem on the infinite level of time and space. This disease is a problem unique to our planet.

Finally, the 'plague' is viewed from a cosmological perspective, as a humble reminder of our responsibility to maintain planetary equilibrium, for humanity itself is a 'virus in the Universe.'

> On the other hand, everything in the universe is in a state of equilibrium. Our creators told us that our planet is just an atom of a gigantic being who is alive and who is gazing at other stars and asking himself if there is life on other planets. The creators told their messenger, Rael, that humanity is a disease of the universe, and that mankind must not progress too far or he will disrupt the balance of this gigantic being we are a part of. Man is *already* a virus in the universe,

and if the viruses in our bodies proliferate too much, then the entity of man will die. In this way we can see the relationship between AIDS and infinity which has been revealed to us by the ELOHIM.

Raelians are at once pragmatic and compassionate in their concern for the rights and care of PWAs. They do not let an infectious and fatal STD cramp their free-wheeling, free-love lifestyle – and yet they do fit it into their philosophy, reinforcing the warnings of a potential planetary disaster given to Rael by the Elohim. Like other new religions, the Raelians congratulate their movement on the wisdom of their alternative patterns of sexuality, which, in their case, have made condoms obligatory since 1976. Unlike the more sectarian, world-rejecting and communal new religions described above, Raelians do not consider AIDS to be very threatening; for them it is neither particularly contagious nor stigmatizing. This attitude corresponds with their world-accommodating stance vis-à-vis the surrounding society.

The Church Universal and Triumphant (CUT)

Elizabeth Clare Prophet is the charismatic leader of CUT, a religious movement founded by her late husband, Mark L. Prophet, in 1958. The membership might be as large as 30,000 worldwide (*Time*, 28 August 1989). Prophet is held by her 'Keepers of the Flame' (disciples) to be a messenger for the 'Great White Brotherhood' of Ascended Masters and a prophet of God. The notion of the Ascended Masters is similar to that of the *boddhisattva* of Buddhism, and was introduced to the West by Helena Blavatsky. While the church's beliefs are eclectic and ecumenical, many of its key doctrines reflect its theosophical origins, and its historical connection to the Mighty I Am movement, founded in 1930 by Guy Ballard. These include the belief in reincarnation, *karma*, a belief in the existence of Masters of Wisdom and a World Teacher Incarnate, and a metaphysical interpretation of the Bible (Lewis and Melton, 1994). Prophet orally transmits messages from higher beings through her 'dictations,' a practice carefully distinguished in a 1989 church pamphlet from 'psychism,' 'spiritualism,' or 'channelling':

'Rather it is the conveyance of the Holy Spirit of the sacred Fire and the teaching of immortal beings who with Jesus have returned to the heart of the Father.'

Born in New Jersey in 1939, Elizabeth Clare Wulf attended school in Switzerland and graduated from Boston University with a BA in Political Science. Then, in 1961, she met her future husband Mark L. Prophet (1918–73). As the result of a mutual recognition that they were 'twin flames' (a Gnostic concept of the spirit possessing a masculine or feminine counterpart conceived out of the same white fiery ovoid), they married in 1963. The following year, Elizabeth 'received Saint Germain's anointing' to be his messenger (Saint Germain is the Ascended Master of the imminent Aquarian Age, just as Jesus Christ was of the Piscean Age).

When Mark Prophet died in 1973, Elizabeth, as his 'twin flame,' naturally inherited his mantle as messenger and prophet. In 1981 she remarried, this time to 'soul mate' Edward Francis, and purchased the Royal Teton Ranch, a 12,000-acre estate in Montana. She also gave birth to her fifth child, Seth, in 1994 at the age of fifty-five.

Prophet's dictations on the topic of AIDS have their place within a chiliastic world-view, best described as 'progressive millennialism' (Wessinger, 1993) and based on the revelations she receives from Saint Germain and other Ascended Masters. She claims Jesus' reign over the Piscean Age is winding up as we approach the year 2000, to be replaced by the Aquarian Age presided over by Saint Germain. The Book of Revelation is to be fulfilled, and as the Spring of 1990 approached, she warned, 'one hundred percent of mankind's accumulated Karma [might] begin to manifest itself on the physical plane.' This was interpreted to mean that the risk of nuclear war would be greater than ever, and this dangerous situation will continue until 2002. Responding to these messages, the church encouraged its members to invest in building fallout shelters, especially in the mountains surrounding the Ranch. In a 1989 pamphlet, 'Actions Speak Louder than Words,' Prophet presents a well-informed and carefully reasoned argument that 'the Soviets have a big incentive to pull off a surprise attack' since 'the United States is unprepared.' The pamphlet concludes, 'I have warned you through Saint Germain's interpretations of Nostradamus . . . If you do not heed the warning, God pity you . . . and the future of Saint Germain's golden age of Aquarius on planet earth.'

AIDS is referred to in an oblique fashion in Prophet's dictation of 8 June 1986, delivered in San Francisco, in which the Virgin Mary, speaking through her messenger, says:

> Beloved Ones, let this . . . be a prayer vigil . . . for the challenging of the last plagues and all who stand as the dweller on the threshold preventing the people from those cures of Light and the natural cures that are owing to them. I speak of the pollution that is dire in the medical profession – the backwardness, the intrigue and the treachery that does put upon the bodies of this people drugs that actually interfere with the genetic strain of the race.

In a 27 November 1986 dictation from Los Angeles, Saint Germain warns the Keepers of the Flame (through the lips of Prophet) of a certain Plague sweeping God's country:

> I speak of the image of woman and of child and the desecration of the body and of the divine polarity of Alpha and Omega that has likewise been desecrated. I speak of the opening of the pits and of the vials of the last plagues and of what has come upon the earth because people have not challenged the diabolical actions of devils incarnate who have brought with them out of the pit these diseases. Knowing full well they were on their way to the Last Judgment they allowed themselves to be consumed by the plague that they might pass into the mainstream of society to affect the children of the light. (Prophet, 1986:216–17)

The church still adheres to Mark L. Prophet's revelation concerning a 'counterfeit race of soulless automatons programmed to control us and our civilization in the ways of death.' In his book, *The Soulless One* (1991), still sold in the ranch's bookstore, he 'unravels a strategy of darkness that has held mankind in bondage to a will not altogether his own.'

The church-sponsored Summit University Forum held a 1989

conference called *The AIDS Conspiracy* which hosted Dr Robert Strecker, Dr Alan Cantwell, and Jon Rappoport. This event was held at the CUT headquarters at the Royal Teton Ranch in Corwin Springs, Montana. Prophet hosts these conferences every summer and publicly interviews revolutionaries in every field who supply the missing dimension to 'news that affects you.' The different perspectives on AIDS in this conference were summed up in the titles of the videocassette of the event: 'Establishment Cover-Up, Pharmaceutical Scam, or Biological Warfare?'

The invited speakers presented their different conspiracy theories on AIDS – which happened to be mutually exclusive. Dr Strecker, who postulates that the AIDS virus 'escaped from a lab,' received the most air time, but it is impossible to deduce, from watching the videocassette given to me by the Ranch's head of public relations, whether Prophet actually endorses any of these theories. Certainly these conferences would convey the disquieting impression to her assembled followers that America the Beautiful is a corrupt and chaotic nation.

The videocassette of the conference records an interesting moment when Prophet departed from her role of charming hostess and intelligent interviewer to utter what might strike the outsider as a weird *non sequitur* (especially if they are unfamiliar with Saint Germain's warning of the 'devils incarnate' and their 'diseases out of the pit'). Elizabeth Clare Prophet suddenly leaned forward in the middle of a discussion concerning the origins of AIDS and, in her cool and elegant manner, asked Dr Strecker, 'Wouldn't you say that this looks like Arch Fiends from Lost Atlantis reincarnated in the labs of Washington, DC?' (The three scientists giggled nervously, exchanged glances and quickly changed the subject.)

While one might expect that the church's recognition of 'soulless ones,' 'devils out of the pit,' and 'Arch Fiends from Lost Atlantis' would result in the demonization of PWAs, Prophet has nevertheless expressed highly supportive sentiments towards them. On a WBEZ interview on 3 January 1993, she announced that a five-day prayer vigil would be held at CUT's annual Easter conference: 'We're praying to God and his angels for a cure and the stopping of the spreading of AIDS.'

Several Ascended Masters have spoken out for PWAs through Prophet's mouth. A certain Jophiel has stated, 'I ... declare war this day against all in government who are not doing the utmost to stop the influx of drugs in this nation, to stop AIDS ... I am alarmed and you ought to be also' (*Pearls of Wisdom*, Vol. 36, No. 10). Two Masters called Purity and Astrea noted a Christlike aspect to PWAs:

> Just look at those who are dying of AIDS. Look at them as though they were the body of Christ emaciated and their eyes glassy; there they lie in pain ... bowed down by their karma ... You see, you either arrive at golgotha ... by the power of your individual Christhood ... or you arrive without having attained your Christhood, wherefore ... you go through the torment and the torture of the damned. (*Pearls of Wisdom*, Vol. 36, No. 10)

Considering CUT's conservative position regarding sexuality, Prophet is surprisingly compassionate towards homosexuals. Members believe in a celibate life unless one is married – and many practise celibacy within marriage as a spiritual discipline. Prophet's disaffected daughter on the *Oprah Winfrey Show* complained that CUT held that oral sex would consign the soul to outer darkness for several millennia. (CUT officials protest this is a highly exaggerated version of their guidelines, and noted that Moira has since reconciled with her mother.) Homosexuality is definitely taboo, although a CUT minister, Reverend Connors, explained this sexual orientation in non-judgmental terms as a possible consequence of an unfinished heterosexual love affair experienced in a previous life. Elizabeth Clare Prophet voiced her concern over the outbreak of gay bashing in Texas (reported in *Vanity Fair*) and organized a Saint Germain Service on 28 January 1995. After members viewed a 14-minute videoclip from *Primetime Live* on gay-bashing in Texas, Prophet declared:

> The brutal murdering of gays is something that is a blight on our nation. We are looking at this so that we can give our invocations for the transmutation of the cause and core of this very great dark-

ness in our land . . . I can feel the souls of homosexuals in this predicament who have died and those who are still living, who cry out to the World Mother for Divine Justice and for protection.

Ramtha

Speaking through the mouth of channeller JZ Knight, Ramtha has held more than 600 public audiences since 1978 in an effort to help awaken the 'gods asleep in a dream called mankind.' Knight was a cable TV subscription saleswoman, but since Ramtha's appearance in 1977 has founded a new religious movement that attracts many spiritual seekers, among them Shirley MacLaine and Linda Evans.

JZ Knight is a pretty, fragile blonde in her late forties, who appears on the stage of hotel ballrooms and undergoes an extraordinary transformation; she moves in jerky steps, speaks in a deep masculine voice, and soon the powerful personality of Ramtha, the seven-foot tall 'Lemurian' warrior with his archaic speech patterns, his weird sense of humour, and his highly original perspectives on life dominates the hall. As Ramtha, she takes on a masculine *persona* and dons white flowing robes and sports baseball caps and boots. Somehow, the well-groomed American woman fades away and a new, remarkable being takes over, compelling many sceptics to accept his presence.

Ramtha made his first appearance one Sunday in February 1977 when Knight and her second husband were experimenting on the power of pyramids to preserve foods. She looked up and saw 'gold sparkles' and through them a transparent bald warrior nearly seven feet tall who announced: 'I am Ramtha the Enlightened One. I am here to help you over the ditch.' Starting with small audiences in her home in Yelm, Washington, Knight began to travel across the country renting hotel ballrooms to hold weekend 'dialogues' where as many as 800 people gather to listen to Ramtha's highly original gnostic philosophy and ask his advice. Prior to 1985 these events were called dialogues because of their question-and-answer format. In early 1985, Ramtha began holding 'intensives' for the purpose of presenting more advanced teachings. Today, the Ramtha School of Enlightenment offers a demanding course of exercises designed to enhance the students' innate psychic abilities (Melton, unpublished manuscript).

On 17–18 May 1986, Ramtha spoke to 800 people on the necessity of becoming self-sufficient in order to survive the impending dramatic changes in Nature. He outlined his apocalyptic vision and his unusual conception of planet earth as a living entity regularly visited by space brothers. Ramtha (1987:35) warns his audiences of an impending apocalypse which could be roughly summed up as 'nature's backlash.' He predicts there will never be a nuclear war – it is rather the earth that poses a threat in its 'evolutionary processes' – and he presented an unusual vision of an earth 'laced with zippers' about to explode into volcanic eruptions, tidal waves, and earthquakes:

> You must understand that your earth is *moving*, it is *changing*, it is *evolving* and becoming grander ... There are zippers all over the earth. Your earth is laced with them to allow the earth's crust to move, to allow the planet to expand ... The earth is recycling itself through what your scientists call 'plate tectonics.' Know what lava is? It is *future ground* ... the plates that have been created at the bottom of your seas are now ... putting pressure on the zipper. Certainly the waves from the zipper's movement are going to do away with many wonderful homes that were built so close to the sea for that wonderful view. (They are going to get a *grand* view!) (Ramtha, 1987:30–1)

Ramtha's recommendations for survival are to invest in gold, move to the Pacific Northwest, stockpile a two-year food supply, and cultivate vegetable gardens. Since Ramtha's audiences have formed no stable community and there is no membership list, it is not known how many have actually followed his advice. However, real estate agents have watched the migration, and estimate the number at '500 to 1,500 people, many of whom are middle-aged women' (Montreal *Gazette*, 14 April 1984).

Ramtha's concept of AIDS is of a 'great plague' brought about by a variety of abuses, all related to Nature and the body. First, he suggests it is Nature's backlash for the misuse of medicinal plants:

> Know you the reason that parts of South America are going to come under siege of Nature? . . . They grow plants [marijuana, cocaine] that were intended by Nature to be an easement of pain for animal life . . . and they are killing the people of this plane with them, for gold . . . But what goes around is coming back. Very shortly there is coming a great plague upon that land and upon the peoples who are misusing this plant. Understand? (Ramtha, 1987:109)

Next, he compares AIDS to the bubonic plague, associating both diseases with low consciousness and religious persecution:

> There was a year in your counting; it was called 1348. And there was a place called Europe . . . There came upon the shores of that continent a horrid thing. This most odious of plagues did not have religious preferences . . . it devoured only those with the attitude of hatred, bigotry, and decadence . . . The plague, called the Black Plague, was a reprisal from Nature against those whose attitude had collapsed below the survival level . . . Well, you have slipped into decadence liken unto that of the year 1348.

For Ramtha, AIDS is an opportunity to cultivate the *gnosis* in the self:

> In 1348, when the plague had finished its ravages, a new consciousness appeared . . . It is the same with this age that you are in . . . The mind will bloom, and the christus in *all people* will come forth – the realization that all people are God. That is the true meaning of the Second Coming of Christ: 'And behold, there came forth a new kingdom and a new earth. And in that kingdom reigns the Christ, forever and ever and ever . . . This is the destiny of your good earth. You are all God. And when gods begin to have inward collapse, so comes what I call the 'War of Valued Life.' There are plagues now upon your land; and from those plagues are growing more plagues. They will never be cured, and they will take from the world one-

third of your population, before the end of your next decade . . .
These plagues aren't something that comes from outer space! *You
created them*! (Ramtha, 1987:136–7).

Ramtha has been attacked by Christian fundamentalist counter-
cultists for preaching antinomian messages. Texe Marrs, TV evan-
gelist and author of a series of anti-New Age books, warns readers
that 'Ram' means goat, the traditional symbol of Satan, and therefore Ramtha is a demon preaching anti-Christian heresies. (Texe
Marrs is the husband of Wanda Marrs, who wrote *New Age Lies to
Women*, in which she postulates that the Goddess of Wicca is the
Bride of the Antichrist.) Another attack was launched by researcher
Jon Klimo (1987) in his book on channelling, where he accuses
Ramtha of being anti-gay. This notion was taken up by the media
and added to their routine accusations of fraud and brainwashing
directed at a 'cult.' In real life, according to Melton (unpublished
manuscript), Ramtha makes no effort to discipline or redirect his
ramsters' sexual orientation or lifestyle at the School of Enlightenment, where many gays participate in the course.

Some of Ramtha's comments on homosexuality and AIDS might
be better understood within the context of JZ's own marital problems. The story of her romance with her third husband, Jeff Knight,
appears in Jess Stern's *Soulmates* (1987). Initially believing Jeff to
be her spiritual counterpart or 'soul mate' with their shared interest
in Arabian horses and spirituality, she was disturbed when he
turned out to be bisexual and was secretly engaged in sexual ad-
ventures among the local gay community. He contracted AIDS and
knowingly exposed her to infection (fortunately, she did not contract it). Disillusioned, Knight began divorce proceedings in the
mid-1980s. Jeff moved in with his lover but withdrew their cash
reserves from the bank, leaving his wife several million dollars in
debt from their failing Arabian horse business. Knight managed
to reconstruct her life, suddenly achieving remarkable success in
the late 1980s, which brought her fame and wealth. Jeff then reap-
peared and took her to court in 1992 for half her rebuilt estate,
claiming it was necessary to support his AZT and other health care
costs. He also claimed that it was not *his* adulteries that had broken

up their marriage, but it was Ramtha who was the intruder, the original 'other man.' He lost the case but continued to contest their divorce settlement until his death in 1994 (Melton, unpublished manuscript).

In a manner reminiscent of nineteenth-century female mediums (Moore, 1977), JZ Knight channels an entity that defends the rights and dignity of women and challenges male hegemony. Ramtha condemns males for their omnivorous sexual appetite and suggests they have brought on AIDS:

> you are now below survival. Your society is into decadence, perversion. You rape your children. Men defile your women. Men molest one another. You brutalize sex, eroticize violence, and you sell fear in the marketplace – and you are *insensitive* to it! Your consciousness has fallen below survival into decadence. When you come back up to survival, the disease will go away . . .

He affects a profeminist stance:

> You women, for so long you have survived because of your uterus, your vagina, and your breasts. Your body has been your survival. Stop giving your bodies away . . . When you learn to love yourself, you will not need to grab hold of someone else to make you happy or to take care of you. Then you are free, independent.

He admonishes men to refrain from using sex as a powerplay, and to show respect for women:

> And men, you don't have to go out and copulate everything to impregnate the whole world! . . . You don't have to spill your seed every day! Every moment you do that, you are dying. You have to master the desire to molest children for a thrill. You must master the desire to molest your brothers so that you feel you have power over them . . . See women as equals, as brilliant gods, just as you are. That *changes* the shadow, the destiny; that allows you to go forward in harmony with Nature. (Ramtha, 1987:138)

Knowing something of the personal trials of the channeller might shed some light on the complex psychological phenomenon of possession and, incidentally, on Ramtha's interpretations of the meaning of AIDS.

The Vajradhatu Buddhist International Church

When the Chinese communists invaded Tibet in 1959, many Buddhist monks escaped into India. Chögyam Trungpa Rinpoche migrated to Europe and began to teach meditation. In 1970 he moved to America and established a meditation retreat, the Tail of the Tiger, in Vermont. The story of this extraordinary man's odyssey in the West is told in his autobiography, *Born in Tibet*, and the history of Tibetan Buddhism in America has been documented by Field (1986). The Vajradhatu International Church is the oldest and largest of the Tibetan Buddhist sects in America and claims around 3,500 members.

In 1986 the headquarters of the movement was established in Halifax. By this time Trungpa had retired from active directorship owing to his declining health, and in April 1987, he died of a cardiac arrest at the age of 47.

In December 1988 the board of directors of the church in Halifax publicly announced that their current leader, Vajra Regent Osel Tendzin, was infected with AIDS and had knowingly transmitted it to his nineteen-year-old male companion. They formally requested that he resign from his teaching and administrative work. Osel Tendzin fled to Boston to avoid arrest and, in response to the local board of directors who asked him to step down, made a public speech to the Boston Buddhist community (January 1990) in which he admitted that he had been aware of his illness since 1985, but was convinced, as a result of a conversation with Trungpa, that he could 'change the karma of AIDS' and that since he was enlightened he could not transmit it to others and expected to 'beat the disease.'[13]

Osel Tendzin was born Thomas Rich in Newark, New Jersey, and had been a disciple of Swami Satchitananda when he first met Trungpa in 1971. He was installed as Trungpa's Regent in 1976, the first American empowered to be a gateway to Vajrayana (tantric) Buddhism as a dharma heir of the lineage. A charismatic teacher and able administrator, he was respected in the church, and his homosexual love affairs were not condemned in a community that held very liberal views on sexuality and was already accustomed to Trungpa's heterosexual philanderings and heavy drinking.

The church's response to this tragic and embarrassing situation was to issue statements supplying the bald facts and to refuse to comment or speculate on the issue. In Montreal, when I requested information, I was told by the director that members had been advised not to talk about it since it agitated their thoughts and interfered with their meditation. The same director did, however, send me an article written by Stephen T. Butterfield for *The Shambala Sun* (Toronto, 1989, Vol. 3), which explores in a sensitive fashion the difficult dilemma of choosing to trust a spiritual master and of distinguishing between 'real' and 'fake' masters. Butterfield begins by asking 'how the Tendzin scandal can be used to deepen spiritual realization.' He reviews Trungpa's impressive and impeccable credentials and the great honour which this enlightened being bestowed upon Tendzin. He emphasizes that choosing a master is a decision to take a risk, that no teacher can 'protect us from the anxiety of chaos,' and that in the end one must bear the responsibility oneself. There is a disparaging reference to Rajneesh, how 'choosing a fake may be much worse than losing all our money to support a cosmic rolls royce collector.' In the end, Butterfield recommends an experiential approach and describes how the sitting meditation that Trungpa taught him has completely transformed his life, enabling him to 'crack open these habits . . . and discover the luminous, enlightened energy frozen within them.'

The terrible dilemma confronting the author and fellow Buddhist disciples is outlined as follows:

> Osel Tendzin was the preceptor who administered my refuge and bodhisatta vows . . . [which] is a commitment . . . [A] bodhisattva is a refugee who has given up even enlightenment in order to help liberate others from suffering . . . [He] also vows not to harm other

sentient beings. Many Buddhists, myself included, were therefore deeply shocked to discover that Tendzin could keep silent about having the AIDS virus and transmit it to unwitting partners. If he could do that, one is tempted to ask, what did he learn from the dharma? Some members . . . feel that Tendzin violated the basic trust necessary between teacher and student; that he acted frivolously in assuming that he was above ordinary human limitations and could not infect anyone else; that he broke fundamental Buddhist precepts against causing harm, and has therefore disqualified himself as teacher.

The question of relating with the teacher in this situation is especially poignant and sharp . . . for one cannot enter the Vajrayana without complete devotion to the lineage holder who administers the vows.

Finally, Butterfield reflects on the meaning of AIDS from a Buddhist perspective:

AIDS is a potent vehicle for examining and deepening one's relationship to passion. Now that it has entered the heterosexual population, it can no longer be viewed as a 'gay problem' – it is everybody's problem. Buddhists are not exempt, and the Vajradhatu board acted promptly and responsibly to alert all of our members and limit the damage. No one but a fool can look on a prospective sexual partner any longer and be unaware of death. We must consider whether sex is worth the risk, and why we are doing it at all . . . We would like to deny our fundamental vulnerability and insecurity, but AIDS tells us that every act of intimacy is like jumping from a plane. If we hear the message, it becomes an invitation to connect with the vulnerability and suffering of all beings.

. . .

Every case of AIDS arises from the total environment . . . There is no such thing as individually caused misfortune. Death is certain and comes without warning. It may come on the road, in the air, and in bed. The egoless world, what Trungpa called 'the vajra castle,' is built on a charnel ground – the bones of hope and fear, the skulls of self and other, the hair and teeth of personal security. To enter the vajra castle, we must die, every moment, all the time. Any teaching that seeks to protect us from the knowledge of the charnel ground is fake dharma.

Regarding AIDS in this light is not a license to spread the disease, or an excuse for dishonesty. It is a guideline for how AIDS, or any sickness, may be used to deepen realization. The dharma teaches us to prevent harm, but also to transform affliction once it has occurred. Appreciating our common vulnerability enables us to give gentleness and care to our casualties, and to avoid compounding the damage by sending our aggression and blame.

Osel Tendzin's deception raised the problem of succession in an organization based on charismatic leadership, and the result has been a struggle between several factions in the Halifax church. First, there is the 'Court,' composed of Trungpa's widow, Lady Diana, and some of the older, wealthier disciples. Lady Diana has recently sold her house, moved to Hawaii, and is promoting Trungpa's eldest son to be his successor. She and other long-standing members feel that the board of directors should resign for reacting several years too slowly to Tendzin's dangerous condition. There are other factions in the church, each governed by its own core group, such as Shambala, which is secular in its orientation, and Dharmadhatu, which provides meditation instruction. Trungpa's disciples are now turning in three separate directions: to other Tibetan spiritual masters, to the guru in self, and to venerating the deceased master, Chögyam Trungpa Rinpoche.[14]

Conclusion

HIV-infected members have had a dramatic effect upon the internal politics of these four groups. Ramtha's 'politically incorrect' teachings on the AIDS plague unconsciously reflected the real-life marital problems between channeller JZ Knight and her AIDS-infected bisexual husband, leading to negative publicity in the popular media. Ma Jaya started out as a meditation teacher and founder of an orphanage school, but as she attracted more and more HIV-positive disciples and comforted children with AIDS, her ashram turned into a pilgrimage shrine 'in this time of the AIDS plague.' In the Vajradhatu and Rajneesh communities, the fearful word 'AIDS' became part of the rhetoric of warring factions, and served as a rationale to exert greater control over the members' lives. Each organization confronted a scandal that began with a deception: a Rajneesh disciple received fake results on her HIV test and a Buddhist leader chose to hide his HIV status while continuing to sleep with his disciples. In Vajradhatu, the unexpected revelation of the Vajra Regent's HIV status and criminal deception has (understandably) resulted in doubts and conflicts concerning the authenticity of the guru's authority and schismatic movements in the line of succession.

For the Rajneesh, obligatory AIDS testing for the entire commune of Rajneeshpuram in 1985 became a metaphor for their alienation from the larger society, increasingly experienced as hostile and threatening. A reading of the *Rajneesh Times*, 1984 to 1985, conveys the impression that as external threats mounted – land and building disputes with the 1000 Friends of Oregon, defamation suits against Rajneesh's belligerent secretary, the bombing of the Hotel Rajneesh in downtown Oregon (see Carter, 1987) – the more space in their internal newspaper became allotted to AIDS-related themes. By 1984 Rajneeshpuram had become a fortress, guarding the walls of its utopia with obligatory searches and AIDS tests for visitors, elaborate hygienic measures surrounding food and sex, coloured beads on the *mala* necklace denoting rank and date of last HIV test. Rajneesh employed a retinue of bodyguards armed with Uzi submachine guns, and intercity telephone calls were wiretapped (Fitzgerald, 1986). The purity rituals practised by Rajneeshpuram residents at this time expressed the city's siege mentality. Prophylactic measures against HIV infection were explained in spiritual terms and employed in ritual context, reinforcing Rajneesh's ideal of the New Man, godlike in his autonomy and purity. The disciple's body became a microcosm of the social body, both bodies connected and controlled by a scrupulous monitoring of their entrances and exits.

The different levels of concern among the new religious movements regarding AIDS, and their assumptions concerning the degree of threat and contagion, seem to reflect their social organization. If one compares the communal with the non-communal groups – in Wallis's terms (1984), the 'world rejecting' versus the 'world affirming' movements – the new religious movements described in this and the previous chapter may be arranged under the following headings:

1. Type of organization (communal, non-communal, semi-communal)

2. Perception of threat (indicated by compulsory AIDS tests)

3. Sexual mores (free love, monogamy, celibacy)

4. Level of conflict with larger society.

Table 2 clearly indicates that the communal 'high demand' movements (i.e., those on *bad* terms with society) tend to insist on HIV tests and see in AIDS a maximum degree of threat. Non-communal groups, or groups such as CUT or ISKCON (which is currently in the process of disbanding its communal structure) do not insist on tests. Three of these groups enjoy relatively peaceful relations with society, and only one (CUT) has experienced intensely negative publicity. Although CUT is probably sufficiently old and large to qualify as a church, allegations of arms purchases have excited media attention, and CUT has been depicted (unjustly) on national TV as the next Waco (the *Jane Whitney Rogers Show*, 'In the Wake of Waco').

To study these new religious movements as paradigms is important for understanding the possible effects of AIDS upon our society in the future. Both the Rajneesh and Kashi ashrams aspire to provide models for the larger society to emulate – Rajneeshpuram showed in 1985 one way to obliterate the threat of AIDS. Interestingly, a leader of the Osho Commune in Poona claimed that those same 2000-plus former residents (minus the defectors) were retested in 1990, and not one of them had developed HIV.

Table 2
New Religious Movements and Their Attitudes Towards HIV Testing

NRM	Type of Organization	HIV Tests	Sexual Mores	Conflict
Rajneesh	commune	yes	free	high
Unification Church	commune	yes	monog	high
Messianic Communities	commune	yes	monog	high
The Family	commune	yes	free	high
Kashi	non-commune	no	celib	low
Raelians	non-commune	no	free	med
CUT	semi-commune	no	celib/monog	high
ISKCON	semi-commune	sometimes	celib/monog	med
Ramtha	non-commune	no	–	low
Vajradhatu	non-commune	yes	free/monog	low

She explained that the strength of testing lay not in the identification of quarantine candidates, but rather in its role as a *consciousness-raising device*. She pointed out that much of the world's population has a nagging dread that it might be HIV positive, but continues its pre-AIDS patterns of behaviour. 'The beauty of testing,' she declared, 'is that that person rejoices in their health and is from then on very conscious to preserve it. I want to know my future lover's status, and will take conscious steps to protect myself. Testing works!'

Kashi also unveils a vision of the future; a way to live with dignity and compassion in a world where the inflicted and the dying outnumber the healthy. The paradigms offered by Rajneesh and Kashi represent opposite extremes, both utopian, with dystopian undercurrents. Rajneeshpuram warns us of the potential abuses of power that come with testing and quarantine; Kashi might be a parody of our passive acceptance of mass death.

FIVE

Race Wars and Ancient Conspiracies

The LaRouchians, The Nation of Islam, The Black Hebrews,
The Ansaaru Allah Community, The Aryan Nations

According to Studs Turkel's 1993 study, the average American is 'obsessed with race.' This chapter explores the new racialist religions, representing extreme and overt manifestations of this widespread cultural characteristic, to see how they define AIDS as an issue of race. Their theologies are built upon black or white interpretations of the Bible or the Koran. Their radical solutions to racial tensions go so far as to propose *apartheid* or eugenics, or to prepare for an interracial Armageddon. A steady stream of listeners, joiners, and defectors are attracted to these emotionally intense, elitist communities where they can undergo the process of deconstructing and reconstructing their own (socially conditioned) racial identity, and try on new, stylized masks of idealized humanity.

The AIDS statements of Black Muslim ministers and Christian Identity Grand Wizards reinforce our theory that AIDS is used to define social boundaries; for racialist religions are acutely concerned with the purity of the blood line, with procreating 'perfect' children, and with erecting barriers of ethnicity. Clear distinctions between male and female are essential to eugenics programs, so sexual ambiguity is not tolerated, and homosexuals become the degenerate product of 'race mixing.' AIDS is used as a watershed, a separating line between the fully human and the subhuman, the 'real' people created in God's own image, and the demon seed or monstrous hybrids.

Racialist religions adopt the threatened response and interpret AIDS as a genocidal plot. Xenophobic reactions to epidemics are written in the lessons of history. The fourteenth-century Flagellants marched through terrified Christian villages fanning racist conspiracy theories in which the Jews were featured as perpetrators of the bubonic plague. Zeigler (1971:191–2) writes that the Jews were charged as follows:

> that by poisoning the wells of Christian communities, they infected the inhabitants with the plague ... some alleged the Jews were working under the orders of a conspiratorial network with its headquarters in Toledo; that the poison, in powdered form, was imported in bulk from the Orient, and that the same organization also occupied itself with forging currencies and murdering Christian children. In subsequent epidemics the Jews were accused of passing around clothes taken from the dead or smearing the windows with an ointment made from the buboes.

Between 1348 and 1349 thousands of Jews were massacred from Carcassonne to Brussels. The Flagellants would arrive at these towns in their bleeding, self-scourging processions, and rush to the Jewish quarter where they led the populace in wholesale slaughter.

The AIDS pandemic has not inspired equivalent pogroms – yet. However, as Cohn observes (1970:285), mass upheavals and insecurity refuel the demonization of the Jew in this as in earlier centuries, and 'the phantom of a worldwide Jewish conspiracy is related to the phantasies that inspired Emico of Leinengent and the Master of Hungary.' Most of the groups in this chapter tend towards anti-Semitism and espouse conspiracy theories on AIDS as a genocidal plot. The Aryan Nations are notorious for their murders of Jews and black schoolchildren, and AIDS has been seized upon as just another weapon in their symbolic warfare. The La-Rouchians in the mid-1980s claimed that AIDS was spread through drinking water,[15] and blame the Zionists (in league with the 'effete, pederastic environmentalist sun-worshippers') for the poisonous spread of heroin and AIDS.

Conspiracy theories of AIDS that point the finger at racial or sexual minorities might be analysed as just another manifestation of the countersubversion ideologies percolating through our society during periods of social upheaval.

Subversion fears have recurred throughout American history, providing food for countersubversion ideologies that have been used to justify the persecution and scapegoating of witches, Amerindians, Catholics, Communists, Mormons, and religious cultists (Bromley, 1991). Fears of subversion, Bromley notes, tend to emerge during periods when there is tension or conflict among contemporary social patterns. Once a central problem is defined, its source is attributed to human agents who are designated as morally inferior. The social construction of extreme moral degradation, he claims, moves the target group to a symbolically distant and alien position, which in turn mandates a repressive response:

> Subversives are depicted as having infiltrated a once secure terrain; initially undetected they have become a . . . rapidly growing presence; they are highly organized . . . ruthless and unscupulous, they possess the capacity for corrupting individuals . . . major institutions, even the entire social order is depicted as in imminent danger of falling prey to subversive domination. (Bromley, 1991:59–60)

Subversion fears are proliferating with the spread of AIDS, stimulating the dissemination of countersubversion ideologies whose stunted forms can be detected in our popular culture – but they find their most luxuriant expression in racialist religions.

The LaRouchians

Lyndon H. LaRouche, Jr, is the product of a New England Quaker upbringing. By way of Marxist economic theory and radical left-wing activism, LaRouche has become the leader-founder of what the Heritage Foundation has called 'one of the most bizarre cults in American history' (Shapiro & Lumenow, 7 April 1986:38). For ten years LaRouche has 'prowled the fringes of establishment politics,' running for the presidency in 1976 and 1980 under the aegis of the National Democratic Party (not to be confused with the Democratic Party).

LaRouche's apocalyptic ideology is an eclectic synthesis of 'neo-Nazism, a passionate demand for more nuclear power and conspiracy theories featuring such disparate personalities as the Queen of England, William Mondale and Jane Fonda' (Methvin, 1986:91). History and contemporary politics are interpreted as a battle between those who favour evolution and salvation through technology, and those reactionary oligarchies and financiers who batten on the masses by advocating solar energy. The latter group he charges with attempting to plunge humanity into primitive social conditions through bringing about equality for women and minorities. Those who advocate the decentralization of power and environmental safeguards are labelled 'effete pederastic environmentalist sun-worshippers.' The key to LaRouche's global strategy is nuclear fusion energy – 2,500 U.S. nuclear reactors by the year 2000 – which would take the country into a free-energy economy. His 'great Design' is to seize control over the United States government in order to forge a global alliance of international LaRouchian republics under whose tutelage humankind will be transformed into a super-race of 'golden souls.' According to Methvin (1986), the LaRouchians' utopia would of necessity exclude the 'bestial mass of ignorant sheep which is 99 and 44/100 percent of the human race.'

LaRouchians believe that 'Zionist' financiers operate through the 'drug lobby' to control an intricate network of banks and criminal syndicates. All through history, the 'Zionist-British organism' has committed monstrous crimes against humanity that range from destroying Greek civilization through 'Asiatic sex cults,' poisoning popes, running slaves, assassinating American presidents, and (most recently) inventing heroin and the AIDS virus.

Lyndon Larouche's autobiography, *The Power of Reason: 1988* (LaRouche, 1987), concludes with some unusual perspectives on the AIDS problem. First, he accuses public authorities of incompetence and deliberate deception in handling the issue:

Our government, and many other institutions of the world, have chiefly been lying wildly about the nature and danger of AIDS. First, as I have said, unchecked spread of AIDS, without a cure or a vaccine, means the extinction of the entirety of the human species within thirty-five to forty years, more or less.

Secondly, he denies that it is essentially a *sexual* disease:

> AIDS is not a sexual disease, but essentially a blood-transmitted disease. The same type of disease exists among sheep, cows, and horses, among other species ... the arguments issued by governments and leading bodies of medical institutions are essentially absurd. [They] have not a single experimental fact to support their claim that AIDS is primarily a sexual disease. (Larouche, 1987:324)

Thirdly, he proposes a three-pronged panacea for the pandemic:

1. public health measures based on identifying the persons already infected,

2. preventing infected persons from spreading their infection to others,

3. a 'crash program' on AIDS and related problems modelled on the Apollo project.

Regarding the third prong, LaRouche feels that research into artificial biospheres, essential for space exploration, is an area that overlaps with research on AIDS. Hence, expansion into space is the way to overcome the 'apocalyptic reality of AIDS':

> The Mars project typifies the positive roadway leading up out of our presently worsening condition, the failure to face the apocalyptic reality of AIDS, typifies the absolute breakdown of presently existing policy-making structures. The link between the scientific work needed for the Mars project, and the scientific work needed as part of the conquest of AIDS, expresses the efficiency of the approach I have outlined, both to build the future, and, simultaneously, to ensure that a future exists to be built. (Larouche, 1987:326)

The LaRouchians also see AIDS as a form of biological warfare, introduced into this country by a Soviet spy. In a 1985 pamphlet, the *Executive Intelligence Review*, Dr Sergey Litvinov was named as the chief perpetrator of the AIDS conspiracy:

> Litvinov personally runs the global chain of command for WHO [World Health Organization] of all international AIDS information and projects. Litvinov, who trained at the Institute of Tropical Medicine in Moscow, coordinates the activities of the Atlanta WHO's Task Force . . . and the West German activities . . . Litvinov is known to be issuing straight Soviet Propaganda such as 'blaming AIDS on the United States.' Details on Litvinov and other shocking aspects of the Soviet angle to the spread of AIDS will appear in the next issue of *EIR*. ('Soviets Are Running the AIDS Coverup!' 1985)

This article accuses the American government of sloppy security measures and warns that 'the AIDS pandemic is deadlier than nuclear war.' The solution urged is as follows:

> Therefore, we propose that the United States now declare a full-scale global war on AIDS in the interests of the security of the Western Alliance. Among the principal features of this war must be the objective of eliminating the disease-spawning conditions caused by the economic-austerity conditionalities policy of the International Monetary Fund in the tropics.

LaRouchians associate AIDS with homosexuality and the liberal attitudes of heterosexuals in the counter-culture. A 1985 flyer, distributed in Montreal in August 1985 by the National Democratic Policy Committee, bears the headline, 'LaRouche Warns: "Spread Panic, Not AIDS." ' The article asserts that AIDS is the most deadly global pandemic since the bubonic plague. It blames the gay rights lobby for blocking the 'growing public demands for quarantine measures to assist in containing the pandemic,' and also politicians who, estimating the margin of the gay vote, 'had often traded away their morals by identifying themselves as defenders of the "civil rights of homosexuals." ' The pamphlet goes on to declare that the anti-AIDS political movement (i.e., the LaRouchians) will make the homosexual threat their 'number one sub-issue.'

> The role of homosexuals in creating the massive concentration of infection, from which the pandemic spreads to other portions of the population, and the strong concentration of homosexuals among such occupations as teachers, medical paraprofessionals, dishwashers, cooks, waiters, hair-dressers, and other service occupations through which contamination is most easily spread. The vulnerability of children to infection in schools, playgrounds, and so forth, will be the sub-issue around which the political fight is being concentrated now.

The LaRouchians' prophecy concerning the ultimate effect of the AIDS 'pandemic' on American society is as follows:

> Politically, the growing anti-AIDS political movement will develop a strong anti-liberalism character. Initially, this trend will center around the fact that legalized homosexuality, the 'sexual revolution' generally, and quasi-legalization of the 'recreational-drug subculture,' are the most widespread social expression of the post-1963 eruption of the 'radical counterculture.' There will be a powerful 'backlash' against the 'radical counterculture' generally, a backlash which will spread and grow as an anti-liberalism backlash.
> The anti-liberalism backlash will have the effect of fostering a surfacing of traditional moral values from among what Vice President Spiro Agnew once called 'the silent majority.' Sizable portions of the sectors of the population caught up in the 'youth counterculture' of the 1960s and 1950s, lacking such traditional moral values, will react to their terror of AIDS, either by causing the burgeoning of radical-right populist (quasi-fascist) political associations, or serving as a recruiting-ground for novel varieties of religious fundamentalism. The political danger is, that if the moderates from the 'silent majority' fail to seize leadership of the government, the new 'radical right' will form a fascist movement to fill the vacuum.

The message is clear: vote for Lyndon LaRouche. He will expose the conspirators and dispel the darkness, rescuing those victims duped by an evil plot to control the world and subjugate the masses.

The Nation of Islam

I am warning you, black people of America and white people of America: The end of America is now in sight. You could save your miserable lives, but you're too filthy and wicked. You hate me for warning you. You hate me for defending another servant of Almighty God, my brother, Rev. Jesse Jackson. Before 1989 comes in, we will close out both books – the Bible and the holy Koran – and the world will be in the throes of that which will destroy every power that is on this Earth in preparation for a new gospel . . .

— Minister Louis Farrakhan

Minister Louis Farrakhan is the leader of the Nation of Islam, one of the most powerful of the post-Garvey religious movements in America. Founded by Elijah Muhammad in Chicago, this sectarian neo-Muslim group seeks to unite American blacks through a theology of the land, a faith in the Divine as a liberating power throughout history, and communal moral values. Elijah Muhammad revealed his racial/millenarian theory as follows:

Allah created the first humans (black) who founded Mecca. A Mr Yacub rebelled and was exiled with his 59,000 followers to Patmos, where they separated into two races through eugenics. The pale race was morally weaker and became a race of devils that brought war and crime to earth. Moses was sent by Allah to civilize the whites who would rule the earth and enslave blacks for 6,000 years. Then Allah sent W.D. Fard to relay his message of the liberation and impending millennial supremacy of the black race to Elijah Muhammad.

Farrakhan was born in New York City and christened Louis Wolcott by his middle-class Episcopalian parents. He was working in nightclubs as a Calypso singer in the mid-1950s when he joined the Nation of Islam and, after Malcolm X defected, became the leader of the large Harlem centre. When Elijah Muhammad died in 1975, his son Wallace Muhammad became the new leader and proceeded to change the direction of the movement towards integrating whites and adopting a more accommodating approach to the larger society. Farrakhan, who had moved to Chicago, then led a schismatic movement to reform a new Nation of Islam closer to the vision of its founder. This excluded whites, made black nationalist demands, emphasized economic self-reliance, returned to stricter dress codes, and re-established the paramilitary unit, the Fruit of Islam (*The New York Times*, 19 November 1988). During Jesse Jackson's presidential campaign in 1984, Farrakhan supported his candidacy and became a leading spokesman for the black community on radio and television and at press conferences.

The Worldwide Church of God (not exactly an unbiased source) complained that the City Council of Washington, DC, had decided to honour Minister Farrakhan for his success in cleaning out the drug dealers from a project called Mayfair Mansions, and summed up the 'paranoid, hate-filled, and downright lunatic delusions' expressed in his Washington, DC, Council Commendation speech as follows:

> the whole Farrakhan message: that white people are a bleached version of humanity – a genetic mistake; that whites are intentionally importing drugs, guns, and the AIDS virus into black neighborhoods as part of a calculated scheme of genocide against the blacks; that blacks are the new chosen people who are going to take over control of the world; and that Farrakhan is going to lead them. (WWCG 1978, April)

Referring to Farrakhan's well-publicized anti-Semitic statements during the Jesse Jackson campaign, the WWCG, as Anglo-Israelites, understandably find it alarming that he describes whites as 'white devils' and Jews as 'the most white of all.'

Minister Louis Farrakhan's views on AIDS were expressed on the Phil Donahue show in 1989:

Phil Donahue: Is it your feeling that AIDS is a manufactured disease that has hit in an especially horrendous way among people of colour . . . and was engineered by a white person?

Louis Farrakhan: It is becoming increasingly clear in medical circles that the configuration of that virus is not a natural configuration, that it is a *made* virus. Now, this should not come as a shock to you because viruses have been used for years to get rid of unwanted and useless populations. I think that General Amherst sent smallpox up to the Indians in blankets, and I think you will find that 400 black men in the Tuskegee experiment were injected with the most virulent form of syphilis and allowed to cohabit with whomever they would and never be treated for syphilis – this is reality! Now we're looking at not only biological warfare, but we're looking at chemical warfare in crack cocaine and now in ice being used on black and white . . . and if America doesn't wake up, your country will be lost from within!

That AIDS is conceptualized as a white man's disease by this black community is demonstrated in the 5 August 1991 issue of the Nation of Islam's newspaper, *The Final Call*, which features a story called 'Into Three Women's Lives, AIDS Enters.' At a meeting in Chicago, 'each of the women told the audience of the need . . . for the Black community to get rid of the notion that AIDS is a white, homosexual disease' (*The Final Call* 10(16):30). Appearing in the same issue is a report of the *Chicago Tribune* article (17 July) concerning French scientists 'unwittingly aided by leading American scientists [who] performed secret, deceptive AIDS vaccine experiments on children in the African country' – because of a shortage of laboratory animals. The article concludes, 'There was no "scientific and ethical justification" for using children, and questions about what happened to them remain' (*The Final Call* 10(16):9).

One of the NOI's most gifted and charismatic ministers, Dr Alim Muhammad, gave a speech (n.d.) on AIDS at the Mosque Maryam in Washington, DC, that was taped on videocassette and has been shown across the nation to the local study circles. A poster adverising the 12 December 1988 showing in Montreal features a cartoon of a leering scientist handing a test-tube festooned with skull, cross-bones, and swastikas to a U.S. General in exchange for cash. It claims: 'Germ warfare at its best with documents and proof. President Carter's World Commission to control population decreed that 2.7 billion non-White people must be eliminated from this planet by the year 2000.'

Dr Alim Muhammad, in his electrifying taped speech, ties the advent of the virus – and its cure – into four key doctrines of the NOI: its creation myth, its emphasis on Africa as the sacred cradle of humanity, its conspiracy theories, and its expectation of an inter-racial Armageddon around the year 2000. He announces that 'it is no accident' that it is in Africa that the cure for AIDS has been found – by Dr Kavey Koech, a Kenyan, who produced the drug Kemron.

It appears that Dr Koech's claim has gathered support. While 'most in the international medical community dismissed [Koech's] research and data,' as Alvin Peabody notes ('NIH to Begin Kemron Drug Test,' *Informer*, 25 April 1996:1), eight years later, 'the National Institute of Allergy and Infectious Diseases in Bethesda, MD is launching a national study on whether Kemron is effective in reducing the symptoms of AIDS,' and is calling for 560 volunteer patients. Meanwhile, experiments on black patients were being conducted under Dr Muhammad's supervision in the NOI's hospital in Washington, DC. A photograph in *The Washington Afro-American* shows Dr Alim Muhammad holding up a sign saying, 'Million Man March: Health Task Force.' On his right stands 'Demetrios Haskins, who is documented as having gone from HIV positive to HIV negative following treatment' (Gilmore, 'HIV Positive? 560 Sought for Kemron Trials,' 27 April 1996:A13).

The Ansaaru Allah Community

Dwight York (b. 1945), known to his disciples as 'The Lamb,' is the founder of the Ansaar movement, which might more appropriately be characterized as not one, but a series of short-lived black-identity movements that derive their symbols and inspiration from

Muslim, Hebrew, Egyptian, and Nubian traditions. He claims to be the great-grandson of the Sudanese Mahdi, whose birth was prophesied to occur in the West exactly one hundred years later. York spent his childhood in Brooklyn, became involved in drug-related crimes in his teens, and spent some time in prison in the early 1960s, where he was introduced to the ideas of Elijah Muhammad. He converted to Islam in 1965, but soon broke away to found his own religion (Philips, 1988:1).[16]

The group's aims, expressed in their literature, are to live a strict Muslim life, to communicate with extraterrestrials, to restore the ancient Nubian race, to raise their children as Nubians speaking Hebrew and Arabic, to survive the coming holocaust, and to separate as a people from the 'Amorite' or 'paleface' decadent culture of America.

The Ansaars' concept of AIDS is closely linked to their idiosyncratic racial theory, a mirror image of white racists' 'curse of Ham':

AL QUR'AAN 18:25
AND THEY REMAINED IN THEIR CAVES THREE HUNDRED YEARS AND ADD NINE (25).
(This passage refers to Canaan, fourth son of Ham and grandson of the prophet Noah. Canaan was cursed because his father, Ham, looked upon Noah's nakedness with 'thoughts of Sodomy' in mind. Consequently, the curse that was placed on Canaan was the curse of leprosy.)

Thus, the Ansaars clearly associate AIDS with the 'paleman' whose white skin, a symptom of leprosy, is a divine punishment for a homosexual impulse.

The myth tells us that after the Canaanites were afflicted with leprosy they fled into the mountains where the cold climate was 'conducive to their leprous condition' and where they acquired the name 'Amorite,' which means 'mountain dweller.' There they 'descended to the level of animals, eating raw carcasses, walking on all fours and mingling freely with ... mainly dog-like animals.' Since 'the salts in their bodies reached a dangerous low, they were unable to reproduce.' 'It was at this point that the lepers were commanded by Nimrod (2311–1941 BCE) to come down from the mountains and kidnap and rape the clean Nubian women of the villages, in order to have sex and produce an offspring that would bear the full curse of leprosy. The mixture produced an offspring with black skin and straight, black hair.' The lepers who remained in the mountains 'fell so low as to mate with the dog-like animals' (As Sayyid, 1990:71–2).

The Lamb notes this disgusting behaviour still occurs among today's 'lepers':

> Presently the act of bestiality seems to be a common trend among the Canaanites (Paleman) wherever you go. You see big French poodles, Great Danes, and Doberman pinschers walking the streets with their female masters. Did it ever occur to you that she was also his sex partner? (As Sayyid, 1990:75)

Another association Ansaars make with AIDS is comets, sent by God to cause plagues:

> Although no one knew exactly how comets caused diseases, men had witnessed the occurrence of major outbreaks of diseases after a comet had passed. An example of this was the Bubonic Plague which struck Europe after the appearance of the comet of 1664. The Black Death as it came to be called, struck down one out of every five persons.
>
> For some people . . . Halley the comet has been around too long and plans for its destruction have been made. For mankind (the Amorite), on earth to attempt to destroy a naturally occurring celestial phenomenon is indeed an evil ambition. The chances of their success in destroying Halley's comet is quite slim. For here, they are dealing with a naturally-occurring phenomenon that is controlled by ALLAHU SUBHAANAHU WA TA'ALA.

The Lamb also advances a more familar conspiracy theory. There are frequent references to Elijah Muhammad in the Ansaar literature, and it is not inconceivable that The Lamb might have borrowed some of Farrakhan's conspiracy theories on AIDS, as the following passages from *The Paleman* suggest:

> There has been much doubt amongst scientists and physicians that the AIDS virus came from Africa. Dr Frances Weising, a Nubian who is a Washington DC based physician, author and lecturer, says she wants to see proof that AIDS is not a man-made disease, since recent information she uncovered strongly suggests otherwise.

Since Africa is the sacred homeland and the site of Eden for Ansaars, it is not surprising they object to the green monkey theory:

> American doctors tried to spread the lie that AIDS originated from the Green Monkey of Africa and spread from the jungle to the city. Again, this is another lie because if this was so, the Pygmies from the bush would have been infected with AIDS first. Research shows they were free from AIDS until infected European prostitutes came to Africa. The World Health Organization (WHO) was also responsible for spreading AIDS throughout Africa when they inoculated thousands of Africans with experimental vaccines.

The infamous Tuskegee syphilis experiment, 'conducted for a period of forty years (1932–1972 A.D.) on unsuspecting Nubian men and their families,' is cited, and its relevance to unmasking the white scientists is noted:

> With this in mind Nubians should not find it inconceivable that the same devilish minded person (paleman) would go a step further and develop a deadly disease that could be spread into the general public, Nubian communities and other undesirable population groups such as the white homosexual population and Nubian drug abusers. (As Sayyid, 1990:232–3)

The Lamb claims that the devil is the 'paleman' and that since the opening of the seventh seal, in 1970, the truth has been let loose, that the rule of the devil will end in the year 2000. He offers as a sign of the paleman's imminent demise the fact that his leprosy is flaring up, exacerbated as he ends his demonic reign on earth. The current advertising for sun blisters, the new threat of skin cancer, the advent of AIDS are seen as symptoms of the last stages of leprosy. If black people catch AIDS, it is because their race has cross-bred with the paleman:

> There are many forms of leprosy that are not openly accepted as such by the medical profession today. These forms are encountered every day and occur among Nubians also because our ancestors are guilty of mixing with the cursed Canaanites. Among these are: Psoriasis, Gonorrhea, Syphilis, Arthritis ... Dandruff ... and, more recently, AIDS. (As Sayyid, 1990:81)

The Black Hebrews

Ben Ammi claims he is the Messiah ushering in the Black Millennium, and defines the black race as the real ancient Jews. He has established a commune in Israel composed mainly of Afro-American immigrants restoring the culture of the ancient Hebrew tribes and practising polygamy. Fervently anti-modern, millenarian, and evangelical, Ben Ammi expresses an egregiously misogynistic theory concerning the origin of AIDS:

> No vessel has undergone so much abuse as that of the woman's body ... after the chemical aerosol sprays and deodorants used externally and the cancerous tampons and douche concentrations used internally. She has had her tubes tied, her ovaries removed, foams sprayed internally, pills swallowed, hysterectomies, mastectomies, caesarians and abortions.

He disapproves of modern woman's efforts to gain control over her own reproductive powers, and his concern is evidently to establish a patriarchal rule over women in his commune. It is interesting that he sees AIDS as essentially a *woman's* disease, transmitted from mother to daughter:

> She has waged war against God and lost ... she rebelled against

Adam and followed the instruction of the devil . . . Disease exists in
the female sex organ at a rate unparalleled in history. Venereal disease has become so pandemic until certain viruses are being passed
on to young daughters . . . Some of these viruses are virtually incurable and, when detected, the women are advised to discontinue
childbearing.

He associates the modern AIDS-contaminated woman with Jezebel
of the Old Testament who, guilty of 'fornication,' was 'punished
with great affliction.'
Following in the footsteps of the other black sectarian leaders,
Ben Ammi accuses the white race of plotting to corrupt and exter-
minate his people:

As humanity heads into the last decade of the 20th century, man
finds himself at a crucial turning point. Man, under the influence of
the Euro-gentile dominion, his mind trained in . . . computor-age
technology is applying his education to the perfection of weapons
of death . . . and of course crack – a derivative of cocaine produced
for Black consumption. (Ammi, 1991:83–4)

At the same time he suggests that AIDS is a divine judgment: 'How
can we see diseases of this sort and not consider them a plague
upon the people?'

The Aryan Nations

The Church of Jesus Christ Christian, better known as the Aryan
Nations, is one of the strongest factions of the Christian-identity
movement in the United States. Reverend Richard G. Butler
founded the church in the 1970s and led his flock from California
to Idaho where he established the twenty-acre Hayden Lake compound. This 'whites only' sanctum is surrounded by barbed wire
patrolled by Doberman pinschers and dominated by a guard
tower. Their tiny chapel is decorated with murals of white knights

slaying serpents and dark people with gorilla heads. The Confederate flag hangs beside the Bonny Blue of Texas and banners displaying swastikas. Initiation involves a medieval knighthood ceremony where young warriors kneel and raise their right arms in the Heil Hitler! salute to Pastor Butler and recite the traditional pledge: 'That which we fight for is to safeguard the existence and reproduction of our race, by and of our nations, the sustenance of our children and the purity of our blood.' Like the Nation of Islam, the Aryan Nations' most successful recruiting terrain is through prison ministry. They currently claim over one million followers in the United States.[17]

The Aryans' racial hatred is directed primarily at Jews (which they spell with a small 'j'), whose origins are explained by Butler as follows: 'The Book of Genesis declares jews to be the progeny of Satan copulating with Eve.' He claims that White Anglo-Saxon Christians are the 'true Hebrew tribes' of the Bible, and that Jesus was a blond Northern European. The Zionist Occupation Government (ZOG) controls the banks, the media, and the federal government, and must be overthrown during the cataclysmic race wars to occur at the end of this century which will herald the Second Coming. All people of colour are 'mud people,' and are on the spiritual level of animals, lacking souls.

The aims of this movement are to balkanize America into white and non-white zones, to prepare for the race wars and extraterrestrial invasions, and to work for the triumph of Christian Identity religion.

The excerpts below were taken from a letter appearing in *Aryan Nations: Calling Our Nation* (no. 52). They were written by J.B. Stoner, a prisoner for life convicted after bombing a school on 19 June 1958, killing fourteen black children. Stoner claims he is the 'innocent White victim of a conspiracy'; that 'anti-Christian Jews' have denied him parole, and he seeks to expose the 'racial nature of the AIDS epidemic,' which the 'Jew-controlled media' are attempting to conceal.

He begins this extraordinary document with a salute to his leader:

Pastor Richard G. Butler,
Praise God for A.I.D.S.!
White Racist Greetings!

He hails AIDS as the 'greatest news event in 2000 years, since My Lord, Jesus Christ and His Apostles were on earth,' and expresses satisfaction in the knowledge that 'with AIDS, God is destroying His enemies and rescuing and preserving His great White race . . . scuttling the black-jewish-queer political alliance that rules America.' He considers AIDS a 'blessing': 'Every day I thank God for His great blessing of AIDS . . . a racial disease of jews and negroes which fortunately also exterminates queers.' He accuses public health officials for covering up the 'racial nature' of the virus ('secret meetings of state officials cannot stop the racial effects'), and claims it is a judgment of God:

> AIDS is the wrath of God. Apparently, God has a strong dislike or hatred for jews, negroids and queers and is tired of tolerating them. With AIDS God is changing society and the political order. The faggots will no longer be able to insult us with their abominations and perversions.

His racial theory becomes somewhat convoluted as he tries to forge links between tribes of the Jews and Africans: 'AIDS/KS was known for half a century as a disease of the Ashkenazic jews who then passed it on to the negroes . . . I have heard no reports of AIDS among the Sephardic jews.' Stoner qualifies his racist message by putting in a good word for Pastor Butler's ally in the cause of segregation, Minister Farrakhan: 'I have prayed to God to spare those negroes who are for the separation of the races and against interracial marriage.' He concludes with a declaration of white racist pride:

Onwards to White Victory!
I'm from Marietta, Georgia!
I shall return!
For Christ and the White Race!

J.B. Stoner,
A White Political Prisoner

Conclusion

The mythic dimensions of racism are evidently alive and well and living in the United States of America. These fantasies of the racist imagination, which conjure up monsters from outer space to intervene in our planetary plagues and race wars, support Goldstein's comment (1987) that AIDS has the 'capacity to reinvigorate ancient stereotypes, not just about sexuality but about race and urbanity.' Indeed, many of the heretical improvisations on Genesis that 'explain' racial differences for white and black racists might have been lifted straight out of Ambroise Paré's *Monstres et prodiges*, published in 1573. This classic work proposes teratogenic theories for the Renaissance mind, and deformities are explained in etiological terms as follows:

1) products of the Devil entering the womb.
2) the introjection of too much/too little semen.
3) mating between a human and an animal.
4) the impression of ugly sights or blows upon the pregnant mother.
(Fiedler, 1978:234)

Other possible causes of monsters include the glory/wrath of God, the mingling or mixture of the seed, the artifice of wandering beggars, copulation during menstruation, and the configuration of the planets.

These ancient 'scientific' superstitions uncannily resemble contemporary theories, such as the green monkey theory or the mixing of semen with blood, and many of our etiologies of AIDS could be updated versions of Paré. Associations with Lost Atlantis, Halley's Comet, the dawn of the Age of Aquarius, extraterrestrial visitors, or planetary disequilibrium are found in New Age groups, UFO cults, tabloids, and horror films. The 'wrath of God' has been adopted as an explanation by televangelists, and we have our own versions of 'wandering beggars' who are both symbols and products of a disordered society.

Fiedler explores the historical connection between 'monsters' and 'race' and notes that as humanistic science gradually demythologized and even obliterated the belief in human monsters, Linnaeus introduced nomenclature such as '*Homo ferus*' and '*Homo monstrous*' and thereby created a new, invidious mythology of race. Some of the racial fears and tensions exacerbated by AIDS reviewed in this chapter remind us of ancient humankind's perceptions of far-off, exotic races as monstrous variations of the human, as demonic, or as part animal. Christian-identity reflections on AIDS as originating among the 'mud people,' or the Ansaaru Allah community's association of AIDS, leprosy, and homosexuality with white skin suggest that the medieval rhetoric of racism has survived on the 'alternative altars' of racialist religions. But racialist fantasies, both white and black, can also be detected in the secular sphere.

Whitman (1991) claims that genocide-conspiracy theorists, who contend that HIV is a man-made weapon developed to destroy blacks, have had 'a surprising resonance' among secular black communities:

A 1990 Southern California Leadership Conference poll of 1,056 black church members found that 35 percent believed AIDS is a form of genocide and 30 percent were unsure; 35 percent believed that AIDS was man-made; 44 percent were unsure.

Distrust of government health programs among low-income blacks can be traced to 1972 when the press disclosed the horrific Tuskegee experiment. It is a well-established historical fact that, starting in 1932, the U.S. Public Health Service tracked the lives of 399 black men who had syphilis and lied to them so they would not get effective treatment. The *American Journal of Public Health* called it, 'the longest experiment on human beings in medical history.' The Centers for Disease Control condemned it as 'akin to genocide' (*U.S. News & World Report*, November 1991:82–4).

'Almost 20 years later,' Whitman (1991:84) writes, 'some inner-city blacks still respond to AIDS prevention messages by invoking the callous Tuskegee experiment . . . anti-AIDS programs . . . have faltered after low-income blacks claimed they were "genocidal."'

One lesson for black youth resulting from Earvin 'Magic' Johnson's sudden retirement due to HIV infection is that 'it could help topple another tenacious barrier: the specious belief that AIDS is a form of genocide,' according to the *Christian Science Monitor* (13 November 1991:7). The basketball star's platform on safe sex is expected to have a powerful impact, for 'heroes like Magic are the embodiment of our youth, our strength and, yes, our imperviousness to death and disease' (*Boca Raton News*, Florida, 8 November 1991:1A). The article concludes, 'perhaps Magic Johnson can persuade more inner-city youths to think of themselves as capable of avoiding AIDS instead of hapless victims.'

The story about Ugandan Charles Ssenyonga, who was brought to trial in London, Ontario, on charges of criminal negligence and causing bodily harm after infecting more than twenty Canadian women with AIDS (Callwood, 1995) is likely to stir up racist prejudice. Headlines such as 'AIDS and Blacks: Risky Sex' (*Emerge*, March 1992) have probably unintentional racialist reverberations. That the advent of AIDS has revived anti-Semitism and supported the plausibility structure of racialist conspiracy theories in marginal religions has been clearly demonstrated. But closer attention to news reports tells us that it has also underscored the lines between black and white Americans and exacerbated racial tensions in the American mainstream.

SIX

Healing Homophobia

Gay Enspiritment in San Francisco, Grassroots Gay Spirituality, New Age Healing Practitioners, Homosexuals in Buddhism

The previous chapters have described religious leaders telling gays who they are and where they stand in the universal scheme of things. Many of their statements could be classified as 'creationist homophobia' (Edwards, 1989). Therefore, it seems only fair to include a chapter on what gays themselves are saying about spirituality and AIDS. This approach departs the from the pattern of the previous chapters, which looked at the responses of pre-existing religions to a still distant and abstract threat. In the case of the gay movement, we find a people already stigmatized for their sexual orientation apparently undergoing a spiritual renaissance directly generated by first-hand experience of the epidemic decimating their community.

The spiritual reflections of homosexuals on AIDS are more complex than the unequivocal condemnation or liberal compassion found in mainstream religions. One reason for this complexity is that the gay movement is not, as Adams and Swaggart would have us believe, a monolithic organization. In this respect it is not unlike the feminist or the black nationalist movements: diffuse, in transition, factionalized, and characterized by ongoing struggles among conflicting interest groups. To what extent it can be said that gays adopt spiritual strategies in coping with AIDS, or are inclined to define the problem in religious terms, depends very much on which individuals, or what caucus in the gay community, one chooses to consider.

It is probably accurate to describe religious homosexuals as isolated in both their identity communities. Within the mainstream churches (with the possible exception of the United Church) they are denied full participation in virtually every denomination and are frequently castigated by religious conservatives. Many leaders in the gay community (which is generally hostile to traditional religious bodies) view gay believer activists as 'dupes and masochists engaged in a neurotic and meaningless struggle' (Hasbany, 1989:21). In view of this discouraging situation, many homosexuals choose neither to struggle for acceptance nor to deny their spiritual needs but turn to alternative conceptions of reality. Therefore, one finds many homosexuals in Buddhism, in New Age groups, in the human potential movement, in Wiccan and neo-pagan covens, and in UFO cults. Gays are frequently enthusiastic participants in new religions that require no more than a loose affiliation from members, make no claims of epistemological exclusivity, and charge fees for training in psychotherapeutic and magical techniques often used for secular ends. Colin Campbell (1972) has dubbed the loosely affiliated network of groups, practitioners, and their rotating clients who share an eclectic mix of occult knowledge and practice the 'cultic milieu.'

The appeal of non-traditional religious groups for gays has, to my knowledge, never been systematically examined. Studies of lesbian-gay occultism suggest that witchcraft groups offer 'ideological solutions to problematic sex and gender roles' (Robbins, 1988:50). It appears reasonable to assume that one would find homosexuals in those new religions that de-emphasize marriage and parenthood and regard the human being as essentially androgynous or spiritually asexual.

Certain scholars are of the opinion that gays do not define AIDS as a spiritual issue, either individually or collectively. Scott Dunbar, a bioethicist who worked with PWAs in the Cleveland Clinic, reports that in his experience, gays are so tired of the judgmental attitudes of mainstream churches that they tend to reject any interpretation of their condition that is not pragmatic or scientific. Stephen Schecter, who wrote *The AIDS Notebooks* (1990), observes that the Montreal gay community was mobilized efficiently to protest police raids on bars, but when challenged by AIDS, 'the community proved to be flakier than the social clamour would have led one to believe, and sex was not the greatest of social glues.' He insists that 'the gay community does not exist.' While this may be the case in Montreal, other scholars claim that the gay communities in New York and San Francisco have responded in caring, compassionate, and practical ways to the AIDS crisis. Paul Schwartz (1989) has argued that the counselling networks, hospices, and mourning rituals provided by the gay community all constitute essentially religious responses to AIDS.

The in-gathering of the gay community in New York includes a religious dimension according to Kayal's thesis because it marks the balance between self-interest and communal involvement that he regards as necessary for self-actualization. He claims the AIDS crisis has forged a link between the private emotional world and the public identity of gays – a process representing a move towards wholeness, and a step away from guilt, which Kayal defines as 'the cleavage of the soul reflecting an incomplete religious journey' (Kayal, 1989).

Schwartz also interprets the gay community's response to AIDS in San Francisco as essentially religious in Robert Bellah's terms, that is, as 'an organized pattern of symbolic forms and acts which relate man to the ultimate conditions of his existence' (Bellah, 1967:19). Schwartz notes the formation of institutional symbolic forms in the founding of Shanti Hospice and the Names Project which embody a religious perspective on the epidemic. The Names Project quilt is an impressive ritual innovation that involves white-clad volunteers unrolling a vast quilt to music and reading out each name decorating the coffin-sized rectangles that constitute a *memento mori* of those who have died of AIDS, sewn by their loved ones. Paul Schwartz argues that the quilt is a totem in the Durkheimian sense, as an outward and visible form, imbued with the 'mana' of a community – in this case 'a clan of quilters, their friends and the presence of the dead themselves rolled up in it' (Schwartz, 1988:19).

Some gay writers and activists have sought to establish a unique homosexual culture that is purified of what they view as the destructive elements in the dominant heterosexual society. In the process, they have embarked on a quest for the authentic inner experience of the homosexual which has often resulted in a self-consciously gay spirituality (Thompson, 1987). Individual homo-sexual artists who have contracted AIDS have produced photo-graphs, prose poetry, and paintings that celebrate the mystical eroticism of a threatened subculture and treat the virus as a met-aphor for apocalypse and transcendence.

Gay sexual expression in the 1970s had a proto-revolutionary, spiritual dimension. Charley Schively of *Fag Rag* affirmed that 'cock-sucking is a revolutionary activity.' The writings of Jean Ge-net and William Burroughs celebrate the existential intensity of the homosexual hunt and the mysterious power residing in erotic states of consciousness. Stephen Schecter writes nostalgically of the vanished heyday of the movement, when it was still a charis-matic community:

> yet there was a time not too long ago when their behavior was emblematic of an entire category of desire for emancipation and self-affirmation. In the seventies public sex was the cutting edge of gay liberation . . . (Schecter, 1990)

Recently, David Wojnarowycz, an HIV-positive gay artist, wrote *Tongues of Flame* (1990; banned in Canada) which exalts the pro-miscuous homosexual lifestyle as erotica and ecstasy 'that allows men to escape, block out and transcend the hell of this life and society.' He interprets the virus as a test of society's compassion and morality and a metaphor for the decay of American culture: 'When I was told that I'd contracted this virus . . . it didn't take me long to realize that I'd contracted a diseased society as well.'

Gay Enspiritment in San Francisco

One of the most dramatic – and highly organized – movements to emerge in the wake of the AIDS epidemic is the spiritual renewal that has been sweeping through San Francisco's gay community since 1985. Don Lattin of the *San Francisco Chronicle* (1989b) wrote, 'In San Francisco the spiritual response to AIDS is a gay response.'

This response is an ecstatic mass movement with an emphasis on faith healing, public confessions or testimonials, and therapeutic collective rituals. Meetings take place in church basements or community halls and are often presided over by gay ex-priests or self-ordained ministers in minority churches. The services may synthesize traditional Christian sacraments with more esoteric rituals, such as channelling and visualization.

These services provide opportunity for emotional catharsis, hugging, and massage. Lattin notes the massage tables crowding the stage at Louise Hay's 'Hayrides' in Los Angeles. An Oakland minister involved in the AIDS Ministry Task Force noticed that the epidemic had affected his mode of anointing the sick and dying: 'I use oil more freely and generously – more like a massage' (Lattin, 1989b).

Some of the meetings show the influence of Alchoholics Anonymous: participants introduce themselves by their first name, declare their HIV status, relate their life story, and often conclude by presenting a problem or soliciting advice from the group. Singing, circle dancing, and 'hugathons' are popular concluding rituals.

There are many testimonials from gays concerning the power of this religious renaissance in the gay movement. Scott Eagleson explains his involvement in Radiant Light (a healing church) as follows:

It's very possible I will die within the next five years . . . I've started wondering what's going to happen to my spirit. It's a pretty powerful little spirit . . . Before AIDS much of the gay community was very superficial, looking for good-looking men and good sex . . . There's still lots of sex in the gay community, but now its safe sex – and there's a lot more love attached to it. (Lattin, 1989b)

James Broughton, poet and filmmaker feels that the AIDS crisis has brought out the intrinsic spirituality of gay promiscuity or 'cruising,' which he valorized in the past as 'the quest for the Holy Male.' He believes the AIDS era has brought out a new awareness of spiritual (as opposed to sexual) ecstasy:

The Holy Male is potentially in every one of us ... A quest for the
ecstatic goes beyond cruising for a congenial sex object ... In the
urgency of our present situation, we should look toward connecting
imaginatively with the souls of our brothers. How else will we become soul brothers? (Thompson, 1987:206)

Reverend Jim Mitulski, Pastor of the Metropolitan Community
Church, noted that two-thirds of the men in his San Francisco
congregation have AIDS. He suggested that this has brought about
a more religious orientation in what has hitherto been a rather
secular-minded church body:

Before AIDS, I never used to talk much about Heaven and Hell,
about death and dying. It seemed like a conservative issue, not a
lively concern for liberal Christians ... But, now ... the afterlife has
become an important spiritual concern here. (Lattin, 1989b)

The gay post-AIDS spiritual awakening might be compared, in
its chiliastic fervour, its ritual innovations, and its collective emotional intensity, to the campfire revival meetings of the Burned
Over District in the last century. The contemporary gay movement
has received relatively little attention, perhaps because it is occurring outside the mainstream churches. A survey of books in the
'gay' section of occult bookshops reveals a fascinating range of
new material on self-healing methods and on the spiritual dimensions of sexuality, written by gay mystics (or healers focusing on
gays) out of their concern over AIDS. These works convey some
remarkable impressions of the ecstatic religion arising out of the
gay community in response to the AIDS crisis.

The impact of AIDS on the gay community has been to polarize
the assimilationists and the radical separatists. While the assimilationists are demanding more AZT, better care for PWAs, and the
effort of their fellows to refrain from those practices that most
offend the straight world, the radicals are turning inward and
searching for a uniquely gay spiritual identity. AIDS has confirmed
the objections each faction has to the other. The assimilationists

believe that the self-indulgent promiscuity of the bathhouses and the S&M subculture has fuelled the epidemic and encouraged the stigmatization of homosexuals. The radicals feel that the materialistic aims of the early movement have turned sour, and that AIDS is a reminder of the true purpose of gay liberation – now finally back on course – moving towards what Don Kilhefner calls 'gay enspiritment' (Thompson, 1987:128).

The spiritualization of the gay movement is not unlike what happened in the feminist movement in the mid-1970s, when books on the Mother Goddess, ancient matriarchies, witches, and the mystical aspects of natural childbirth began to appear. While one could argue that any major cultural movement, as it broadens and deepens, will very likely undergo a spiritual or psychoanalytical phase (what some historians might trivialize as a 'quiescent' phase), it is perhaps not a coincidence that both movements developed spiritual interests during those few years when their participants confronted life's most compelling mysteries. For feminist baby boomers embarking on pregnancies in their late thirties, it was facing the trauma of giving birth. For body-conscious gays in the late 1980s, it was living with a disfiguring and fatal disease.

There is considerable controversy within the gay community concerning the remarkable proliferation of spiritual healing circles, therapeutic self-help groups, shamanic exorcisms, 'channelling,' and meditation workshops in the wake of the AIDS epidemic. These tend to derive their symbols and inspiration from non-Christian sources, which include eastern religions, the human potential movement, Amerindian religion, and New Age. That these alternative spiritual traditions are rising to the occasion and accommodating the psychic and social needs of stricken homosexuals has received ambiguous responses. Relatives and gay friends of the afflicted clients have expressed relief that their loved ones have found a source of support and hope. On the other hand, more cynical friends and secular-minded gays are inclined to dismiss spiritual healing practitioners as snake oil salesmen opportunistically preying on the weak, the desperate, and the rich. Tony Porcelli, a gay activist and pianist whose ex-lover, Ralph Hall, was the sole author and editor of the 1970s newspaper *Faggots and Faggotry* described his perceptions of the religious hysteria sweeping through Greenwich Village today as gays panic before the onslaught of AIDS:

You see all these guys walking around the village and they look really sick and they're wearing all these crystals around their necks, or some of them have got Walkmans and they're listening to Louise Hay tapes all day. And in the gay newspapers you're always seeing ads for healing groups where the guys sit around and hold hands and send out the virus into space. Or you see all these miracle cures and diets that guarantee to restore the immune system and promise all your symptoms will vanish in a week. One of my friends was into this stuff – pond sludge – it's called SPIRULINA, and you send away for it and it's incredibly expensive. He used to mix it up with egg white every morning in my blender . . . Then there is this stuff called 'Compound Q' – it's from a root that grows in China and is supposed to bolster your immune system, and it costs a fortune. I heard a story about a group of gays who chartered a plane and flew to China to dig it up – but untreated it's very toxic, and they got really sick, and a couple of them died. New York is totally polarized now. Every time you open the *New York Times* you read about gay bashing, which is now more popular than ever, and then you go on gay marches and the Mayor joins you! And you see all these famous people walking round the Village, and you feel like you know them because you've read all about their life and you appreciate their work – but you don't really know them. Then you see one of them looking terrible and you say, 'Oh, no! Even he's got AIDS!' Then there's this macrobiotic guru – I forget his name – and he claims if you follow his diet he can cure you of AIDS. He gives appointments where he sits in his office chair, smokes cigarettes and gives out individual diet sheets. I had this friend who was taking care of an ex-lover who was dying and complained that it was all really expensive, and the friend had to buy a whole new set of pots for cooking. Then he got sicker and weaker, even though he followed the diet, and on his deathbed – literally five minutes away from death – he asked my friend to bring him a glass of orange juice, which he really craved. Somehow the macrobiotics people heard about this and they kept phoning up my friend and screaming, 'You killed him! If you hadn't given him that orange juice, he'd be alive today!'

Larry Paradis, co-founder of the AIDS support group New Friends, complained in an interview with Don Lattin that 'a lot of people are getting very rich off AIDS . . . People like Louise Hay are visualizing all the way to the bank . . . I know people who have died because they left the medical world to take vitamins, read every book, and listen to every tape . . . That scares me' (Lattin, 1989b).

The Reverend Matt Garrigan, who founded Radiant Light Ministries and Eternal Life Enterprises, admits that his ministry brings in around $20,000 a month, but protests: 'I really believe what I'm teaching.' His healing practice is rooted in the New Thought tradition of the early 1900s, which stresses the origin of all matter (including dis-ease) in thought. Garrigan updates its nineteenth-century rhetoric with an upbeat patter apparently borrowed from Werner Erhard, promising his method will 'empower you to uncover and convert the blockages you created to experiencing freedom of choice, change, and certainty . . . (Lattin, 1989b).

A critique of Garrigan's flamboyant style was written in the *San Francisco Sentinel* by gay journalist Robert Julian, who presented Garrigan's emotionally overwrought sermons as a gay parody of Jim Bakker. Julian complained in an interview with Don Lattin:

When someone tells homosexuals they are perfect in God's eyes and no one can judge them, a lot of people are going to listen . . . But, will they be able to see through the facade of New Age charlatans and recognize the old money-power game simply manifesting itself in a new form? (Lattin, 1989b).

Porcelli and other activists are likely to view the faith that gay PWAs show in spiritual healing as evidence for AIDS dementia. However, faith healing has been known to work on occasion, and one must commend the courage of those whom the medical profession has pronounced terminally ill, but who continue, like Dylan Thomas's father, to 'Rage, rage against the dying of the light.' Moreover, it is unfair to dismiss all spiritual healers as money-grubbing quacks. Many of the religious leaders who have opened hospices and are conducting Buddhist meditation groups for sick PWAs are underpaid (or unpaid). Some of them (like Buddhist monk Issan Dorsey) are HIV positive. Whatever their initial motivations might be, they are providing a valuable service to the growing community of AIDS patients, gays and straights alike.

Grassroots Gay Spirituality

Gay writers and visionaries since Walt Whitman have created neologisms, constructed new evolutionary theories, and excavated gay histories in an effort to define the essence of that otherness which is 'not heterosexual.' Whitman saw homosexuals ('adhesive people') as possessing spiritual gifts (Moritz, 1987:131). Sociologist Edward Carpenter (1987) argued that 'intermediate types' in primitive societies played important roles as shamans, priests, healers, and artists. Gerald Heard developed a theory concerning the evolutionary function of 'isophyls'; he argued that homosexuals, owing to their prolonged youth, are capable of learning and growing long after their heterosexual age peers have settled down in families and specialized jobs. Hence, isophyls are able to make important contributions to culture (Heard, 1987:176). Coming out in the American counter-culture in 1977, Harry Hays and Don Kilhefner organized the first Spiritual Gathering of Radical Gay Faeries in the desert of Arizona, where participants were invited to 'tear off the ugly green frog skin of hetero-male imitation to reveal the beautiful Fairy Prince hidden beneath.' According to Kilhefner, these trailblazers were dedicated to 'completely redefining ourselves, our history, and our culture outside the Myth of the Homosexual and beyond gay assimilation' (Thompson, 1987:128–9).

AIDS has posed a challenge to gay spirituality in that it has intensified negative attitudes to homosexuals, and many gay writers have reacted by attempting to validate different forms of homoeroticism as essentially spiritually motivated. Others have responded by blaming the advent of AIDS on 'straight' society. Examples of attempts to fit AIDS into gay tantrism, shamanism, millennialism, and psychoanalysis are found in the writings of Mark Thompson, Don Kilhefner, James Broughton, Geoff Mains, and Roger Lanphear (in Thompson, 1987).

James Broughton's 'Enspiritment'

James Broughton, filmmaker, poet, and 'subversive Buddhist,' defines 'gay' as the ability to participate in the transcendental dance of life. Therefore, in his view gay identity is not a sexual nor a social state, but a metaphysical one. There is a millenarian edge to his vision of gay men's role in history. He blames the rape of the earth and the prevalence of warfare on heterosexual consciousness ('Look what the heterosexual ethic has done to the earth with its shameless greed and its passion for war.') He criticizes the materialism and *embourgeoisement* of assimilationist gays and states that homosexuals who cultivate 'gay spirit' have the potential to be world saviours:

> Most gay activists are concerned with what society can do for them. They want acceptance, they want to be absorbed into the social fabric of the heterosexual mainstream. We should be considering what *we* could do for *them*, how we could free them from their misery and wrongheadedness.

Part of gay men's role in their world-changing mission is to remain young and light-hearted 'Peter Pans':

> We are the Peter Pans of the world, the irrepressible ones who believe in magic, folly, and romance. And, in a sense, we never do grow old . . . The gay spirit is a young spirit. That's why the world needs us. We refuse to become dowdy and dull, we refuse to dwindle into the doldrums, and we never die. (Thompson, 1987:205)

He observes that it is very difficult for 'the golden boys' to handle the responsibilty of AIDS. He calls the disease a 'plague, an eruption, an avalanche,' and its function within the evolution of gay spiritual culture is as follows:

> AIDS is an epidemic that threatens all of mankind. Its cause, I believe, derives from the obscene polluting of the earth that exploitative greed has practised. The growth of cancer as a killing agent was the beginning of this poisoning. Now we have a second terrible result of inhabiting a poisoned world that destroys our immunities. Gay men are in the vanguard of this tragedy, they are martyrs to the sickness of their destructive society. We all hope their suffering may help the finding of a cure that will save the rest of mankind. What would be most rewarding to their memories: if they effected a real change of heart in the body politic. Theirs is not a situation of the purely accidental, any more than it is some vengeance of Jehovah visited upon sinners . . . Everything is connected; everything is part of the dance; and everything, alas, is part of the evil that men do. The victims of AIDS are the victims of their warlords and industrialists. (Thompson, 1987:206)

Don Kilhefner and Mitch Walker of Treeroots

Drawing upon the Jungian approach to dream analysis, a small group of men in Los Angeles called Treeroots engages in the on-going task of 'gay soul-making.' Founded by Kilhefner and Walker in 1981, this group explores their dreams in an attempt to reclaim a 'gay-centered spiritual tradition.' In a group interview, conducted by Mark Thompson (1987), members of Treeroots expressed the notion that AIDS was a hint that it was time for gays to turn inward, to 'come out inside' and seek for lasting, spiritual values rather than social acceptance.

> *Mark*: I think the horror of AIDS has served as a trigger for a lot of gay men, signalling that something is obviously not right in their own society, but also on the planet as well . . . Outer reality tends to reflect the inner one. For instance, if, in the past we have characterized gay life as being self-absorbed, superficial, victimized . . . this is a reflection on an inner state . . . AIDS has hastened the awareness

that perhaps gay culture . . . was heading for some awful kind of distress.

Don: The concept of a 'homosexual' – a person whose total identity is shaped and defined by the sex act – is a relatively recent formulation in the Western world . . . And today, with the AIDS crisis, we are reaping the tragic harvest of that mistake . . . We've been participating in a gigantic hoax.

Mitch: The idea of talking about the unconscious as being the shadow is not a bad one . . . The shadow has already come to the gay community, death has come to the gay community in living color! No one can stop AIDS at this point, you see. But it can be related to and worked with just like the unconscious. That's another way of talking about this 'coming out inside' . . . It would be healthy for gay men to . . . discover and develop a real, inner gay world.

Mark: We've been treated as if we were a virus within the body politic of America itself, rather than as an indispensable part of its social fabric. (Thompson, 1987:241–2)

Geoff Mains and 'Leather Magic'

Geoff Mains has written an apologia on the more esoteric mating habits of the gay leather subculture. He labels their sadomasochistic rituals as 'leather magic' and explains their spiritual function as facilitating a shamanic descent to the underworld and inducing altered states of consciousness in its adepts. He claims that some of these controversial homoerotic practices can bring about a spiritual regeneration in the participants and that S&M bondage can create a special bond of trust between participants. He courts the sympathy and understanding of the straight world, seeking to allay their 'suspicion of leather experience' – and even asserts that if more people were involved in it, the world would be a better place:

Now, more than at any other time, those who use leather to explore transcendent experience need its revitalization, its special magic and its powers. In courting these, leather people have something to give both themselves and a world thriving on distrust and disbelief. The heart that screams ecstasy through pain/pleasure speaks directly to its soul and God. The body, immobile in the peace of bondage, momentarily clears its burdens and gains new strength ... This magic carries participants to the edge of their experience and their limits in the manner of shamanic journeys. In achieving this magic, individuals are required to give and trust and be humble. These are all things, perhaps, we could learn more of today. (Thompson, 1987:99)

Roger Lanphear's 'Spirexuality'

Roger Lanphear describes himself in *Gay Spirituality* (1990) as a San Francisco lawyer in the 'establishment' who secretly inhabits the gay world. He is also an inhabitant of the cultic milieu and works as a therapist who combines Transcendental Meditation techniques with Reiki massage, Mahakari light, and channelling. He outlines his 'spirexuality' exercises, which both tap and affirm the spiritual dimensions of sexual experience. In his occasional work as a channeller and healer he has imparted his revelation concerning the millenarian significance of AIDS to several of its victims. He describes how, in the midst of performing 'hands-on healing treatments' to a group of HIV-positive gay 'saints,' he received a 'personal yet universal' message for one of the 'stunningly handsome' men:

> Mark ... you are to know you are on a very significant and divine mission right now. It won't be easy, and you knew when you volunteered ... Just know that you are right on course, doing a profound thing for the earth. (Lanphear, 1990:137)

A few months after, Lanphear met a young dancer with AIDS at a Sunday afternoon garden party, and again 'received my signal from the Master' with the impulse to share it:

> John, we have come here for a special purpose mission. Earth is not

really our home now, but it used to be. There is so much . . . negative energy here . . . some of us are allowing our bodies to absorb it. Then, when we have a full load, we drop the body. It's a really profound thing we're doing, and you're on the front line. (Lanphear, 1990:138)

Lanphear confesses his own trepidation upon going in for an HIV test: 'Could I cope with a positive result? . . . With all of my metaphysical training and those wonderful spirexuality exercises down pat, I still don't know how I would react.'

Lanphear's *Gay Spirituality* (1990) combines UFO lore and Lost Atlantis mythology with New Age apocalypticism, and the result is a theodicy of AIDS that makes martyrs out of gay PWAs and awards them a key role in ushering in the millennium. His revelation for 'a certain number of gay men, lesbians, and a few enlightened heterosexuals' is that they have been reincarnated many times on earth, but in the latter days of Atlantis escaped to Egypt and Mexico in order to 'preserve the sacred knowledge' and 'crystal power.' When even these outposts fell victim to spiritual darkness, this group moved to another solar system. Planet earth is presently entering a critical moment in history and 'the possibility for a new dawning is here,' the awakening of humanity. To this end, 'billions of souls from other unenlightened planets and star systems have converged here. Their own Higher Selves knew of the possibility to discard forever the chains of ignorance' (Lanphear, 1990:126–7). In order for this to be realized, however, 'much negativism needs to be neutralized. Vibrations need to raised several octaves.' One of the ways for gays to dissipate negativism is to 'use our bodies as sponges. We let our bodies absorb negativism, even to the point of illness. AIDS is one such illness . . . It is like cleaning up chicken litter, using our bodies as wipers. We wouldn't have agreed to this if it wasn't absolutely necessary' (Lanphear, 1990:132).

Planetary 'negativism' also includes 'deadly wars, thinning ozone layers, nuclear waste, cutting down the rain forests' and other environmental catastrophes. The fatal consequences of contracting AIDS are also explained: 'If we keep absorbing negativism into our bodies . . . we'll reach the saturation point and drop the body. We see this happening all around us, and to say it isn't easy is the understatement of the millennium.' The Master, channelled through the author, assures this 'incredible group' that 'we have come as the road crew to pave the way for an enlightened age,' thereby 'fulfilling our mission as enlightened lesbians, gay men and enlightened heterosexuals' (Lanphear, 1990:142). Finally, Lanphear encourages his gay and lesbian Atlanteans to look on the bright side:

> Yes, this disease is life's most difficult time for many of us . . . Neutralizing negativity is not for sissies. We're shovelling up all the crap that's been building up for eons. It must go, or humankind will end up destroying the planet and God knows what else with it . . . It is such a privilege . . . to help usher in the enlightened age! . . . Let's always try to remember that there is indeed perfection. Even AIDS fits into a perfect scheme, and it can only be for the good. (Lanphear, 1990:140)

New Age Healing Practitioners

The New Age has responded to the AIDS crisis with upbeat messages packaged in books and courses on how to heal oneself. One interesting example is Nick Bamforth's *AIDS and the Healer Within* (1987). The author offers the reader ten meditation exercises based on the seven chakras, or nerve centres, which are located along the spine and are described in terms of their relation to the coccyx and the pineal gland. Various emotions such as guilt and bereavement must be explored and exorcised through visualization exercises and affirmations as the afflicted reader works through the book and up the spine towards health and spiritual realization.

While a footnote assures us that 'this book . . . can be used in harmony with traditional medicine,' its professed aim is to 'teach how each and every one of us is able to assume total responsibility for our own health instead of passively relying on traditional medicine to find a cure for us.' The author blames the medical profession and the press for insisting that the disease is fatal, and claims that 'in putting forth their own limited and negative understanding of AIDS' they are depriving PWAs of the inner strength to fight the disease.

Bamforth states he has known many people whose lives have been enhanced and become more meaningful as they faced the challenge of AIDS, and many have achieved a 'relatively stable condition.' The message of AIDS on an individual level is as follows:

> For so many people I know, myself included, AIDS has been the stimulus to recognize this higher reality within us and to cast aside all the superficial crap that we have allowed to clutter up our lives. In confronting a potentially fatal disease, we are led to confront our deepest selves. If we fail to do this, we are running away from our own source of strength, the Healer Within. (Bamforth, 1987:6)

While this book is not written specifically for gay men, the author includes a chapter on 'Homosexuality and AIDS' in which he commends gays for their 'questioning spirit' and for following their own instincts in the face of social censure. He notes that the two impediments to healing or 'negative factors' frequently encountered have been parents' rejection of gay sons and religious bigotry. He urges homosexuals to release their sense of underlying guilt fostered by their religious upbringing, and to recognize God within, whose essence is love.

On the planetary level, Bamforth explains that AIDS is a catalyst to prepare certain people for this 'change in energy' leading to the birth of the New Age. He defines the New Age as a 'fundamental shift in Consciousness' and the end of the Old Age, the Age of Pisces. Christ the Fisherman was the herald for the Old Age and his oft-misunderstood message, like that of other great prophets and healers, was 'God is Love' and 'God is Within You.' This message has been perverted by the Catholic Church which 'spends all its energy on sin and guilt' and by fundamentalists who 'preach a regime of intolerance and self-righteousness.' The New Age, however, is a 'renewal of that spark of . . . True Christ Consciousness' which will enable 'Mankind and the Earth . . . [to] raise themselves out of the power chakra into our rightful place of the fourth chakra, the centre of the heart' (Bamforth, 1987:140).

From a New Age perspective, therefore, the eschatological significance of AIDS is the following:

> On a global scale, AIDS is symbolic of changes, the birth pains that the Earth is going through. AIDS is a disease . . . primarily rooted in the third chakra, the centre of power and strength. To rise out of it, we must leave power behind and open our hearts to love in its broadest sense. This is exactly what the Earth and Humanity must and, indeed, will do.

Louise Hay and the United Church of Religious Science

Louise Hay is a New Thought minister in a religious tradition founded by Ernest Holmes in the 1940s. In tandem with his brother, Fenwicke Holmes, he sought to synthesize the inherent truth found in Christian Science, Hinduism, Whitman, and especially Thomas Troward. They created Religious Science, which emphasizes the power of thought within a psychological system that equates spirit with Universal Mind (God) and the subconscious mind of Man. The human subjective mind, therefore, contains God's creative power, but acts upon suggestions from the conscious mind to cause either health or disease (Judah, 1967).

The relevance and the comfort that this philosophy offers PWAs is easily understood. There need be no fear of judgment in the afterlife, since God is love. Through making mistakes and suffering in this world, humankind will wax in spiritual knowledge and will continually progress. Rejecting the notion of a transcendent God who enters history, Religious Science believes in a God who is immanent within each human being, as the following passage from their creed illustrates:

> We believe in the incarnation of the Spirit in man and that all men are incarnations of One Spirit . . . believe in the eternality, the immortality, and the continuity of the individual soul, forever and ever

expanding . . . believe the Kingdom of Heaven is within man and that we experience this kingdom to the degree that we become conscious of it. (Judah, 1967)

'We believe in the healing of the sick through the power of the mind' is also stated in their creed, and since all diseases are rooted in thought (Christian Science), and are subject to cure by reorienting the mind and its thoughts, the notion of an incurable disease runs directly counter to their beliefs. (Melton, 1989: xxi)

In spite of the evident appeal these doctrines have for PWAs, Louise Hay is one of the few ministers in Religious Science who is willing to take up the challenge of AIDS.

Hay's healing approach is presented in two books, *The AIDS Book* (1988) and *You Can Heal Your Life* (1987), and she can be heard on audiocassettes conducting 'treatments,' which Religious Science defines as 'the process of changing our minds to conform to God's goodness.' She explains that AIDS is caused by society's and parents' negative attitudes towards homosexuality which her clients have grown up with and have internalized as feelings of guilt or self-hatred: 'It is my belief that venereal disease is almost always sexual guilt . . . It is not surprising that gay men were amongst the first to experience the deadly disease, AIDS' (Hay, 1988:136). Healing AIDS, therefore, is a two-step process that involves first, 'stop criticizing yourself' and then 'learn to love yourself,' which the following 'Deservability Treatment' helps to achieve:

Deservability Treatment

I am deserving. I deserve all good. Not some, not a little bit, but all good. I now move past all negative restricting thoughts. I release and let go of all the limitations of my parents. I love them, and I go beyond them. I am not their negative opinions, nor their limiting beliefs. I am not bound by any fears or prejudices of the current society I live in. I no longer identify with limitation of any kind.

In my mind, I have total freedom. I now move into a new space in consciousness, where I am willing to see myself differently. I am

willing to create new thoughts about myself and about my life. My
new thinking becomes new experiences.

I now know and affirm that I am one with the Prospering Power
of the Universe. As such, I am now prospered in a multitude of ways.
The totality of possibilities lies before me. I deserve life, a good life.
I deserve love, an abundance of love. I deserve good health. I deserve
to live comfortably and to prosper. I deserve joy and happiness. I
deserve freedom, freedom to be all that I can be. I deserve more than
that. I deserve all good.

The Universe is more than willing to manifest my new beliefs.
And I accept all this abundant life with joy and pleasure and grati-
tude. For I am deserving. I accept it; I know it to be true.

Hay goes on to argue that the emphasis on youth and beauty in
the gay subculture has resulted in a lack of respect for the inner
person. She lists some of the aspects of the gay 'destructive lifestyle': 'the meat rack, the constant judging, the refusal to get close
to another, etc. are monstrous. And AIDS is a monstrous disease'
(Hay, 1988:137).

While appearing to celebrate the pursuit of homosexual freedom, Hay questions the motivations behind the promiscuous bathhouse lifestyle:

The bath houses fulfil a wonderful need, unless we are using our
sexuality for the wrong reason . . . we are getting bombed out of our
heads every night, if we 'need' several partners a day just to prove
our self-worth, then we are not coming from a nourishing space.
We need to make some mental changes. (Hay, 1987:138–8)

Marianne Williamson and A Course in Miracles

Another New Age practitioner who offers gay PWAs spiritual
solace, if not the hope of recovery, is Marianne Williamson, described in *Vanity Fair* as 'not only the guru of the moment in Hollywood . . . but also a leading spokeswoman for a quasi-religious
phenomenon that is making waves around the country' (*Vanity*

Fair, June 1991). The 'phenomenon' to which they are referring is the best-selling book *A Course in Miracles*, which outlines a system of spiritual training. This book was not written, but 'dictated' between 1965 and 1972 through the late Helen Schucman 'by a source she became convinced was Jesus.' Williamson and other spokespersons promote and direct over a thousand study groups in the United States in a 'self-study program of spiritual psychotherapy.'

Both the doctrines and Williamson herself seem to hold a great appeal for gays and PWAs, and *Vanity Fair* suggests that:

Many people see the anxieties of the age of AIDS as a primary explanation for the growing popularity of *A Course in Miracles* which asserts that all human beings are innocent and carries none of the judgmental sting of Christianity. (*Vanity Fair*, 1991:174)

In 1987 Williamson founded the Los Angeles Center for Living, which provides free meals, house cleaning, counselling, and massage for people with 'life-challenging illnesses.' The New York Center for Living has since opened, and another charitable organization, called Project Angel Food. It is staffed by volunteers delivering over two hundred meals a day to home-bound sick people in Los Angeles. Williamson's charities are fashionable in Hollywood and in the New York art scene. Movie stars attend her lectures and help prepare the meals; her star-studded board of advisors includes Kim Bassinger and David Hockney. Besides delivering public sermons on *A Course in Miracles*, which are praised as showing deep insights into contemporary problems, Marianne Williamson leads a monthly HIV-positive support group in New York. She responds to the psychic and physical problems of participants with 'compassionate but tough' advice, 'all with the spiritual underpinnings of *A Course in Miracles*.' She leads the group in prayer and comforts them with her conviction in the immortality of the soul: 'Physical incarnation is highly overrated: it is one corner of universal possibility. The life-force cannot be destroyed.'

Homosexuals in Buddhism

The Buddhist response to AIDS in America is an important element in the gay community's spiritual response to the crisis, presumably for the reason that Gordon Melton offers in *The Churches Speak on AIDS* (1989): 'Many homosexual people turned to Buddhism which offered a less judgmental approach to their personal sexual orientation than they had found in traditional Christianity' (Melton, 1989:174).

Two Buddhist organizations offer hospice and care for dying PWAs and encourage them to explore traditional Buddhist teachings on suffering, death, and dying. Meditation classes for PWAs are offered in California and Vancouver in which many of the participants are gay and long-term meditators. These various Buddhist organizations include the Buddhist AIDS Project in Richmond, California, founded by Ken McCleod; Living in Each Moment, a meditation class founded by Kristin Penn; and the Hartford Street Zen Center's Hospice, founded by Issan Dorsey.

Buddhist Meditation and AIDS

Kristin Penn is the editor of a journal of Buddhist meditation called *Karuna*, which is published in Vancouver. In November 1987 she decided to offer a meditation class for people with AIDS and ARC, and wrote a report of the class in 1989 featuring interviews with four of its nine participants. These contain testimonials on how the group support and Buddhist meditation has inspired them to live the time they have left with greater awareness, and to accept their impending death calmly.

Penn describes the format of the group as follows:

> I had no preconceived notion of what the group would be like . . .
> We meet in one member's apartment and begin the group with each
> of us saying how we are feeling. Then we discuss a topic . . . what
> does forgiveness really mean? How can I learn to live with pain?
> What did the Buddha mean when he said we could be free from
> suffering? . . . half an hour of discussion, we meditate for forty

minutes: 30 minutes of Vipassana (insight meditation) and 10 minutes of Metta (loving kindness) ... we might have a special meditation on hearing, using sounds in the environment and the sound of bells. After the meditation we have tea and informal conversation.

The testimonials that follow are quite moving as expressions of courage and affirmations of spiritual life. They appear to be written by four highly cultured and articulate homosexual men who state that contracting the virus has given them the opportunity to put Buddhist principles into practice, to distance themselves from the career rat race, and to focus their consciousness on the present moment.

They each affirm the value of community that the group has provided:

I also wanted to be part of a group of men and women who shared my belief in the importance of spiritual life. I felt a need for sangha ... where none had existed hitherto. In this group, I have felt my heart begin to open. (Sean)

When I first came ... I was astonished by how accepting the group was ... 'You're perfectly okay the way you are' ... began to realize I was a full, multidimensional person and was reminded of all the things I wanted to be and do that I had suppressed. (Jerome)

They talk about how they understand their homosexual orientation within the context of Buddhist philosophy:

After returning to Canada, I began the process of acknowledging and expressing my homosexuality. This process was one of both celebration and difficulty. The Buddha talks about having to work with our desire, hatred, and ignorance. Well, for the next ten years I became heavily obsessed with desire, desire that did not take into account that I also had spiritual needs. ... This whole self-created melodrama had begun to wind down before I took ill with AIDS ... (Sean)

The spiritual meaning they derive from AIDS is an enhanced ability to live moment to moment with an immediate and sensual awareness of the world around them, a state of consciousness akin to the Buddhist model of enlightenment. This ability appears to result from facing death:

> The circumstances of having a life-threatening illness have forced me to look at the world differently. . . . I see the world more closely and with others could see it that way as well. We're all in such a bloody rush – to Armageddon, it would seem. I like to just sit and watch the birds come and feed at the feeder outside my window. (Bill)

> The last few years before I was diagnosed with AIDS I was getting more and more ambitious, working on an accounting degree which was just going on and on forever. All that came to a screeching halt. What a relief! My priorities have completely changed. This may sound a little lofty, but I feel like what is most important for me right now is learning to love . . . I always thought I wanted to leave the world a better place than I found it, but I thought that meant building something or doing a work of art. But I realize now that if you can introduce some love into the world, what better thing can there be to leave? I may never get to build a bridge . . . but I can spread some love. There's a lot of time for that. (Richard)

> The idea of having AIDS and being 'doomed' to some short-term future doesn't really worry me any more. The first issue I raised in the group was about facing one's mortality and dealing with the fear and anxiety involved. After a short time, being here and alive right here and now became much more fascinating. (Jerome)

(*Karuna: A Journal of Buddhist Meditation* 6(1) (Spring 1989): 13–19)

Issan Dorsey and the Hartford Street Zen Center

The late Issan Dorsey (born Tommy Dorsey in 1933) is a remarkable example of spiritual influences in both the gay movement and the counter-culture. A former female impersonator who was an enthusiastic participant in the beatnik era, during which he shot speed, then partook of the bathhouse scene of the early gay movement, and later joined the hippies in dropping acid, he finally sought refuge and sanity in the San Francisco Zen Center under Roshi Richard Baker in 1969. Issan Dorsey served as head monk of the the Big Sur Monastery for many years but, on receiving a positive HIV test, decided to move to the smaller Zen centre in the Castro section of San Francisco in 1987 to open a hospice for sick and dying PWAs. He and his Zen monks and students acted as nurses, counsellors, and meditation instructors to their patients and viewed their work as a *sadhana*, leading them to a deeper realization of the Buddhist doctrines on suffering and impermanence. In an interview with Don Lattin of the *San Francisco Chronicle*, Dorsey commented, 'AIDS is like a slow earthquake . . . We've slowed the earthquake way down and have an opportunity to watch the dying process. That's a great gift.' He also observed that he had always sensed a strong spiritual impulse in the gay community which was often misdirected into drugs, alchohol, and sex, but now AIDS has prompted gays to 'accept their life as it is and start taking care of each other' (Lattin, 1989a).

Conclusion

The remarkable responses reviewed above are convincing evidence that gays are just as inclined as anyone else to spin metaphors out of the dark cocoon of a mysterious disease. Gay images are not so different from those found in 'straight' groups: it is a 'plague,' a 'slow earthquake,' a 'shadow,' but its moral or meaning is not the same. The notion of a divine punishment or judgment upon homosexuals is, of course, strongly denied. Rather, AIDS is often associated with society's unjust persecution of sexual minorities, and some New Age healers even go so far as to suggest that sexual guilt and homophobia has actually engendered the virus. Other gay visionaries explain AIDS as just one of the side effects of a poisoned and exhausted natural environment. They blame this sorry state of affairs on the patriarchal heterosexual culture which has always sought to dominate and devastate nature, women, and peace-loving men. A few gay prophets see the epidemic as serving a millenarian purpose, and award stricken gays with a salvific role as martyrs and vital actors in ushering in the new millennium.

It is tempting to interpret the more extreme heterophobic theodicies of AIDS in political terms, as mirror images and defensive reactions to some of the more obnoxious homophobic chiliasm of televangelists and others. On the other hand, these theodicies make sense in psychological terms as 'a search for meaning in the face of a devastating plague – a crusade to experience life fully in the face of the unrelenting march of death' (Lattin, 1989b). Whatever explanation one chooses to accept, it cannot be denied that gay spirituality has forged its own brand of metaphorical thinking about AIDS and that these metaphors serve to define and protect the boundaries of the gay community. First, they create a sense of distance and separation from their accusers and judges. Broughton, for example, has turned the tables on homophobic Christians by accusing them of polluting the earth and poisoning the mind, unwholesome conditions which gave birth to the virus (Thompson, 1987:200). Secondly, these metaphors serve to reinforce a feeling of unity and brotherhood among homosexuals. Support groups such as the Mastery Course or Roger Lanphear's channelling circles appear to provide a rite of passage for gay PWAs, enabling them to come to terms with their new social and physiological status, to rearrange their priorities, to bond with fellow sufferers, and to establish new perspectives on their own bodies. Some healing circles appear to foster in their members a self-conception as saints and martyrs: Lanphear's clients would presumably take pride in their world-saving mission as elite Atlanteans, and meditators in Buddhist *sanghas* express the feeling that they are more fully alive and conscious than they were prior to their illness.

Gay spirituality experiments with the body and reorders its symbols. A photograph of the Gathering of Radical Faeries shows a circle of shaggy men, their naked bodies coated in mud, grinning and embracing ecstatically, presumably about to 'tear off the ugly green frog skin of hetero-male imitation to reveal the beautiful Fairy Prince hidden beneath' (Thompson, 1987). Geoff Mains de-

scribes the autoplastic rituals of the leather subculture which transform the human body into something resembling an insect larva
or a spider's wrapped prey:

> Eyes, face and neck are wrapped in black leather and laced up the
> back; there are holes for the nostrils and mouth. Then, to complete
> the enclosure, John puts his own jacket on David, zips up the front
> and handcuffs him behind the back . . . A harness made of leather
> that is used to subdue horses is strapped about David's waist . . . as
> chains . . . attached to rings in the ceiling and walls, the body it
> contains will eventually slant forward and then float free.

Mains insists that the aim of this exercise is transcendence or
'apotheosis':

> this bound body speaks ironically of peace and freedom . . . The
> strength of a human body frozen in its glory. Bondage in its fullest
> is no mere pastime. Like all forms of leather, bondage can be apoth-
> eosis. (Thompson, 1987:107–8)

Other gay writers see the homosexual body as expressing eternal
youth. James Broughton calls his gay brothers the 'golden boys,
the Peter Pans of this world.' Roger Lanphear channels the image
of a gay, sick body as a 'sponge' inhabited temporarily by an
immortal Atlantean to mop up 'negativity.' Thus, in the gay social
body, one finds a familiar determination to control the exits and
entrances of the physical body. One finds the same conviction that
many religious bodies feel: that by blocking up or stimulating the
'five senses' and closing or enlarging the orifices of the body; by
pruning sexual energy, or letting it cascade freely, that it is possible
to control the congress between the social body and the surrounding society, and (what is more relevant for the religious individual),
it is possible to awaken to the spirit tappings from the world within.

SEVEN

A Virus in the Popular Imagination

PWA Portraits, AIDS-as-Monster in Cinema, AIDS:
From Anomaly to Anomie

PWA Portraits

The fear of AIDS outstrips the fear of other diseases, for it is rooted in the fear of the Other, the alien, the profane.

People with AIDS are feared because they are perceived as perching on the fuzzy line between the living and the dead, the male and the female, the respectable and the depraved. Thus there is an ongoing tug-of war between the compassionate desire to reclaim them as fully human, and a primitive desire to reject them as wholly alien. The stigmatization of HIV carriers has been characterized as a facile strategy adopted by the mainstream in order to avoid the trouble of reassessing its own heterosexual and hygienic habits. Goldstein of the *Village Voice* makes this point in his article about the expanding social categories for its candidates in New York City: 'As the boundaries of infection extend, more and more of us will live in fear of being stigmatized. And in the end . . . the whole city will bear the brand of AIDS' (Goldstein, 1987). The author, who is gay and sensitive to the process of stigmatization, has even observed this strategy operating in his own mind:

Every time I heard about another death, I would strain to find some basis for a distinction between the deceased one and me: He was a clone, a Crisco Queen, a midnight sling artist. Then Nathan died of AIDS, and Peter, and Ralph . . . There is a secret logic we apply to people with AIDS: They are sick because they are the Other, and they are the Other because they belong to groups that have always been stigmatized . . . In the Bronx today, six percent of women over 25 using a prenatal clinic . . . test positive for [HIV] antibodies. Are they junkies? Are they faggots? Are they niggers? Are they us? (Goldstein, 1987:17)

John Platt (1987:10–15) echoes this point: that AIDS, in jumping from group to group, is following the pattern of other exponentially growing epidemics in the past, for 'each group thinks of those caught earlier as being a wild and wicked minority, and it congratulates itself on escaping until it is suddenly overwhelmed in its turn.'

A study of PWA portraits that have appeared in magazines from 1985 to the present is an interesting exercise in observing the expanding and contracting margins of deviancy, as the population of the virus's victims relentlessly increases. The subjects of these portraits range from famous film stars to pre-pubescent haemophiliacs, to African wives, to gay S&M connoisseurs, but in each case the task of the journalist is to redefine and clarify the boundaries between what is 'normal' and what is deviant; what is fully human and what is monstrous. The important concern underlying the following PWA stories, therefore, is to establish to what extent the person afflicted is 'just like us' and to what extent he or she is deviant or 'Other.'

Deviance, as Berger (1969) and Scrambler (1991) define it, is a property of the social order conferred upon those individuals who are perceived as threatening the boundaries of the symbolic universe. The deviant become identified with the recurrent intrusion of anomic phenomena such as evil, suffering, and death. Two kinds of social deviance are identified by Mankoff (1971): *ascribed deviance*, meaning the unearned stigma attached to the ontologically offensive citizen such as the mad, the blind, or the crippled; and *achieved deviance* or rule-breaking. PWAs fall into either, or occasionally both of these categories. AIDS-stricken gays, blamed for their behaviour, are relegated to the achieved category, whereas haemophiliac children bear no more than the faint aura of ascribed deviance that surrounds the dying. Many media biographies of PWAs take on the task of *improving* the protagonist's status by raising it from achieved to ascribed deviance, e.g., showing how the virus was contracted from a blood transfusion, rather than from homosexual activity. The journalist's next step is to embark on the process of 'deviance disavowal' (Goffman, 1968). This involves establishing a 'fictional acceptance' of the PWA as normal, breaking through prejudices and working to sustain a definition of the person as fully human. Some stories 'go with the flow' of society's deeply ingrained prejudice against homosexuality, for they protest: 'This guy isn't gay, so don't reject him.' Other stories are more confrontational, telling us: 'This guy *is* gay, but gays are beautiful, innocent human beings too!'

A deviance disavowal story is *People* magazine's cover story on Ryan White, a sixteen-year-old haemophiliac who 'in the shadow of death . . . has found a great gift of living. This is a boy you will never forget.' The story simultaneously stresses his normalcy and his heroism (*People*, 30 May 1988). Another example of this strategy is the depiction of AIDS patients in popular daytime soaps. Deborah Rogers (1988) complains that, although *Young and Beautiful*, *All My Children*, and *Another World* have received accolades for addressing a significant social issue, 'they have in common one disconcerting element: all three AIDS plots on these television serials feature patients who are women – and women with no history of drug abuse.' Moreover, all female characters are involved in ongoing romantic – and sexual – relationships (one even marries a millionaire after she is diagnosed). Rogers finds this worrisome:

> While I am not suggesting that people with AIDS should be denied love and understanding, AIDS might seem inappropriate for a character in romantic fiction, especially since the implications could be seen as dangerously misleading for viewers . . . And there is another possibility that is far more distressing. I think it is fair to assume – unless we are explicitly told otherwise – that marriages are consummated. If the message here does not endorse sexual intercourse for people with AIDS, what does it convey?

These sentimental portraits of PWAs are not unlike the consumptive heroines of romantic novels and fiction in the last century, and they might be interpreted as guilty overreactions to the fear and loathing of PWAs in the public sector, telling us, 'Look, PWAs can be romantic and heroic, too. Let us reclaim them as fellow humans.'

Portraits that cannot fail to underline the 'otherness' of PWAs are the stories following the deaths of Rock Hudson, Way Bandy, Robert Mapplethorpe, and long-time survivor Michael Callen.

Rock Hudson

Rock Hudson's death from AIDS in October 1985 was a small but signal victory in the long struggle to legitimate homosexuality. The actor went to great lengths to keep his illness secret and appeared to be more concerned about his romantic image than his own life. 'I hope to die of a heart attack before they find out' was his initial response to his diagnosis in 1984. Confronted with the dilemma of a kissing scene in *Dynasty* and having to choose between possibly infecting Linda Evans or harming his career, he 'ducked the decision.' His biographer, Sara Davidson, wrote, 'Rock used every gargle, mouthwash and spray he could lay his hands on,' and the infamous kiss turned out to be 'a dry peck on the cheek.'

Rock also neglected to inform his live-in-lover, Marc Christian, about the diagnosis. However, the situation turned out happily for the young man. A Los Angeles jury awarded Christian $21.7 million in damages from Rock Hudson's estate, and he has tested negative several times. Christian has since announced his intention of trying to establish a 'serious relationship' with a woman.

Ironically, once Hudson's health collapsed and he entered a Paris clinic, he was hailed for his 'courage' and 'honesty' and became a martyr in spite of himself. Elizabeth Taylor mounted a star-studded benefit show in his honour to raise one million dollars to fight AIDS. President Ronald Reagan phoned to wish him well. Rock received thousands of telegrams and letters from fans who clung loyally to their idol's macho image on the silver screen. After Rock, AIDS could no longer be shrugged off as a distasteful minority phenomenon, but had leaped from the ghetto to the 'glitterati,' and this was a boon to fund-raisers. As *People* magazine (1989, Fall:Extra) summed it up, 'it seemed impossible that one man's fatal infection could transform the public image of AIDS from a four-letter word into a shared emergency. But it did.'

Way Bandy

Way Bandy was a famous and fashionable make-up artist in New York in the late 1970s and early 1980s who died suddenly of AIDS in 1986. An elegant sprite of a man, he was so enamoured of Georgia O'Keeffe that he once hired a limousine to drive him from Manhattan to her ranch in the desert of New Mexico. True to her reputation as a recluse, she refused to see him.

The report of his illness caused some alarm among models and socialites because of the close-up contact his art demanded. He claimed that he never licked his brushes as he applied make-up to his subjects' lips and eyelids, but dipped them in pure spring water.

Way Bandy was the quintessential self-created man. A former married high school teacher in Alabama, he left his wife and moved into the high-fashion world of New York:

By that time (when he arrived in New York) he had already become Way Bandy ('The name just came into my consciousness'), having shed the name with which he had been born in Birmingham, Alabama. He never revealed his true name ... he was several years older than his official age ... He wanted, in his words, 'a new beginning,' and he proceeded to remake himself, with the new name, a nose job, a new hairline, and a new livelihood.

Bandy was evidently a participant in the 'cultic milieu' (Campbell, 1972):

Bandy said he was aware of previous lives, and confident about living more. He said he was 'evolving his spirit' to become the most enlightened person possible by using the powers of the mind ... Bandy could impose his will to make things happen. Taxis, for ex-

ample. He would just . . . stand a few feet away with his eyes shut
. . . and that damned Checker would show up, heated and with good
music.

Like the Rajneesh, Way Bandy was a vegetarian and washed all
his vegetables in bleach. He was aloof, independent, and autono-
mous. A homosexual, he gave up sex (unlike the Rajneesh) as soon
as he heard about AIDS. The identity of his parents remains a secret
contained in sealed court records. His ideas on the family might
have been learned at the knee of Bhagwan Shree Rajneesh: 'Families are just an accident of birth . . . They're just a conduit to get
here.'

The moral of Way Bandy's story is clear. He strove for greatness
and perfection and achieved it. He was famous, wealthy, handsome, beloved by his chic friends. His clients included Nancy Reagan and Tina Turner. In the end, however, he fell from greatness,
betrayed by a double-headed nemesis: his need for sexual intimacy
and his inability to erase the past. AIDS has often been described
as 'a blow to the sexual revolution.' Perhaps it is also a blow to the
cult of the individual, and heralds the demise of Tom Wolfe's 'Me
Decade.' AIDS is a hidden weakness, acquired during a brief, existential moment of passion; a seed planted unwittingly in the
forgotten past. AIDS is the nemesis of Lasch's 'new narcissist'
(1978) who, liberated and self-absorbed, believes it is possible, in
Werner Erhard's language, to 'create your own reality.' For Way
Bandy – and disciples of Rajneesh – AIDS becomes a metaphor for
the failure of the modern human being to reconcile conflicting
needs for intimacy and for autonomy.

Robert Mapplethorpe

Robert Mapplethorpe, the controversial art photographer, declared, 'For me, S&M means sex and magic, not sadomasochism.
It was all about that.' He is described in Dominick Dunne's (1989)
article in *Vanity Fair* as 'the man who had taken the sexual experience to the limits in his work, a documentarian of the homoerotic

life in the 1970s at its most excessive, resulting, possibly, in the very plague that was killing its recorder.'

Mapplethorpe was released from St Vincent's Hospital to attend his own vernissage at the Whitney Museum in July 1988. The article in *Vanity Fair* features 'before and after' pictures of the artist, first at twenty-five, a faun-like, mischievous beauty, and more recently, as he appeared at the Whitney:

> He was in a wheelchair, surrounded by members of his entourage, carrying a cane with a death's head top and wearing a stylish dinner jacket and black velvet slippers with his initials embroidered in gold on them – a vastly different uniform from the black leather gear that had become his trademark. His hair looked wispy. His neck protruded from the wing collar of his dinner shirt like a tortoise's from its shell. But even ill, he was a man who commanded attention, and who expected it.

The *Montreal Mirror* described Mapplethorpe as an 'unapologetic fag' whose work was a 'testament to gay hedonism' which 'documented and helped define a sociology of modern love' (*Montreal Mirror*, 22–29 March 1990). His importance as an artist and martyr to AIDS appears to reside in his recording of a gay subculture. Whereas the practices he portrays would probably be considered depraved and incomprehensible by most Americans, because the subculture they represent is literally dying, these rituals are no longer seen to pose a serious threat to American mainstream values, and yet they are sufficiently remote and exotic to count as art. An anonymous rival photographer interviewed by Dunne commented, 'The smart society that has accepted his work has done so because it is so far removed from their own lives.'

Mapplethorpe seemed to possess the shamanic ability to travel between two worlds and, in dying, to bring the two worlds together. Portraits of bejewelled society ladies such as Paloma Picasso and Caroline Herrera hung beside leather-strapped men engaged in silent, esoteric acts of humiliation. Somehow this artist had succeeded in stretching the boundaries of taste and moral tolerance. It wasn't that S&M had become tame, even for sophisticated New Yorkers. Dominick Dunne states, 'However much you may have heard that this exhibition was not a shocker, believe me, it was a shocker.' But suddenly, for some reason, homoerotic S&M was chic. This could be seen as a breakthrough for certain segments of the gay liberation movement: 'People in the Circle [the highest category of membership in the Whitney Museum] . . . came up and said they thought it was wonderful the Whitney was hanging the show.' On the other hand, the show could be seen as a moratorium on the liminal phase of the gay sexual revolution. Dunne notes the reactions of viewers at the vernissage:

> They went from I-can't-believe-what-I'm-seeing-on-the-walls-of-the-Whitney-Museum looks to nudges and titters . . . to a subdued sadness, a wondering, perhaps, of how many of the men whose genitalia they were looking at were still alive.

The *Montreal Mirror* refers to Mapplethorpe's photo exhibition as 'nostalgic' and an *in memoriam* that 'captured the sense of abandonment and exploration that marked the gay world . . . in the '70s. Before the advent of AIDS put a damper on all festivities.'

Mapplethorpe attempted to articulate the moral and aesthetic dimension to controversial practices such as fist-fucking, urolagnia, coprophilia. As he explained in the interview with *Vanity Fair*:

> Most of the people in S&M were proud of what they were doing. It was giving pleasure to one another. It was not about hurting. It was sort of an art . . . For me, it was about two people having a simultaneous orgasm. It was pleasure, even though it looked painful.

Mapplethorpe, the man, resembles Way Bandy as a self-created aesthete who rejected his family ties to redesign his life from scratch. He shares the same passion for order:

> Mapplethorpe's rooms revel in the pleasure of art for art's sake and reconfirm his aesthetic genealogy in a direct line from Oscar Wilde and Aubrey Beardsley through Christian Berard and Jean Cocteau . . . But everything has its place. Order and restraint prevail. 'You

create your own world,' said Mapplethorpe. 'The one I want to live in is very precise, very controlled.'

Mapplethorpe is the artist-hero whose indomitable will manifests itself in moments of physical strength: 'On the opening night this amazing strength came to Robert . . . At the end of the evening he got up and walked out, after he had come in a wheelchair.' He was also a philanthropist who left part of his considerable fortune to AIDS research. He was a pioneer in the rather rarefied field of black homoerotic S&M photography:

> He once said, 'At some point I started photographing black men. It was an area that hadn't been explored extensively . . . I found that I could take pictures of black men that were so subtle, and the form was so photographical.' Now, musing on that, he said, 'Most of the blacks don't have insurance and therefore can't afford AZT. They all died quickly, the blacks. If I go through my *Black Book*, half of them are dead.'

There is a dark moral in Mapplethorpe's success story. It is a Dorian Gray story in reverse: as his horrid artworks become more beautiful with exposure, so the artist himself ages prematurely with a disfiguring disease. Perhaps the public's rather ghoulish fascination for his work lies in the fact that, in many of these carefully posed photographs, he might have documented the exact moment of the deadly virus's passage from one body to another. Seen in this light, the photographed figures in the Whitney represent a grim dance of death, or a visual journal of a plague.

Michael Callen

Michael Callen rejoices in being the longest-term AIDS survivor on record: 'There isn't any rational language for me to describe how I feel. All the imagery is religious or spiritual. I feel blessed. I feel lucky. I can't believe I'm still here.' He was still alive and doing well nine years after a diagnosis of full-blown AIDS in 1982. The portrait of Callen by Celia Farber (1991) in *Spin* is complex and full of contradictions.

The founding father of the 'PWA self-empowerment move-ment,' he is a living testament to the power of positive thinking:

> I'm not saying all you have to do to survive AIDS is have the right attitude. But I have found, time and time again that those who give up – who say to themselves, 'Death is inevitable, so why fight it?' – they seem to go very quickly. Whereas the fighters, who say, 'God-dam it, I'm not going to let AIDS control my life!' – they hang around a lot longer.

Callen challenges the notion that AIDS is a fatal disease:

> All of the long-term survivors I interviewed believe in the possibility of their own survival ... They refuse to buy into the media's unre-lenting message of doom and gloom ... For most people, AIDS is about dying, but for some people it's a challenge to start living.

This PWA credits Dr Joseph Sonnabend with saving his life. Son-nabend has devised a 'multi-pronged' approach that creates a med-ical safety net which, for Callen, involves taking up to fifty pills a day of preventive medications. AZT is rejected, however, as 'in-compatible with life.'

A heretic within the gay movement, Callen was once one of its most outrageous participants. When asked by journalists how he contracted AIDS 'he would flash his bright green eyes and say quite matter-of-factly, "By the time I was diagnosed with AIDS, I calculated that I had had at least 3,000 people up my ass." ' Rein-forcing 'straight' stereotypes of gay sex as unhealthy and dirty, he would confess to the formidable array of sexually transmitted dis-eases he had contracted in the past. After working with Dr Son-nabend, and possessing an experiential knowledge of gay lifestyle, he has concluded that the breakdown in the immunity system is a 'sociological problem ... the unimaginable amounts of sex com-bined with recreational drugs resulted in repeated infections and other immune-suppressive factors, ultimately leading to the immune collapse known as AIDS.'

Callen has written two books, *How to Have Sex in an Epidemic* (1990) and *Surviving and Thriving with AIDS* (1988), which criticize the gay-liberationist rhetoric that proclaims that sex is inherently liberating and hence, by a 'curiously naive calculus,' assumes that more sex – with more partners – is more liberating. Callen came to the conclusion that, 'Unwittingly, and with the best of revolutionary intentions, a small sub-set of gay men managed to create disease settings equivalent to those of poor third world countries in one of the richest nations on earth.' For this reason, Callen urges gay men to reform their sexual habits: to stop being promiscuous and to avoid the exchange of bodily fluids. His first article in 1982 (co-authored with Berkowitz), called 'We Know Who We Are: Two Gay Men Declare War on Promiscuity,' sent 'shockwaves' through the gay community. Published during the heyday of the gay sexual revolution, it was interpreted as a 'self-flagellating guilt trip.' Gay author Edmund White's contrasting statement was popular with radical gays of the period: 'Gay men should wear their sexually transmitted diseases like red badges of courage against a sex-negative society.' Callen's warning was so unpopular that 'People walked up to me on the street and spit in my face' (Farber, 1991:20).

Callen's unorthodox views are contradicted in other ways. His damning critique of AZT has offended AIDS activists who are pushing for its greater availability. He also pokes fun at the sanctimonious posturing of some PWAs:

> There is a tendency for some people with AIDS to bludgeon people with their disease. People lose sight of the fact that having AIDS does not make you automatically a good person. It doesn't make you holy. If you were a shit before, chances are you are going to be a shit as a PWA. (Farber, 1991:21)

When asked by reporters how he has managed to live so long, Callen would joke, 'Luck, Classic Coke, and the love of a good man,' or would quote his mother's opinion, that he's 'too mean to die.' He draws on the metaphors of an advanced technological society to express his experience as a PWA:

> I hear this stewardess in my mind say, 'We are beginning our descent. Please fasten your seat belts.'
>
> . . .
>
> AIDS is a roller coaster ride without a seat belt.
>
> . . .
>
> It's like standing in the middle of the New York Stock Exchange at midday – buzzers and lights flashing, everyone yelling, a million opinions, a momentum . . . (Farber, 1991)

Callen's strategy to combat AIDS is a mixture of positive thinking, 'empowerment,' preventive medicine, and an open mind to whatever seems to work. As he admits himself, 'I've made it my mission to share confusion . . . because that's all we have.' While his cynical sense of humour struggles to de-mythologize some of the 'New Agey' approaches to healing ('This isn't some est seminar!'), at the same time he offers testimonials to the power of the spirit to overcome disease: 'AIDS has taught me the preciousness of life and the healing power of love' (Farber, 1991).

What Callen's example has achieved is to establish a new image for PWAs. Since AIDS is generally held to be fatal, PWAs tend to be regarded with a mixture of pity and horror; as still alive but marked for imminent demise. They are seen as neither truly alive nor yet quite dead, but dwell somewhere in the twilight between these two states. Callen contradicts this image by having led an extremely active and creative life for over a decade. As Farber notes, 'He has more energy than you or I.' Through his example he has forged a new identity for PWAs: as sick people, much like diabetics, who are responsible for their own health and capable of living extended, productive, and meaningful lives.

AIDS-as-Monster in Cinema

Cinematic depictions of global destruction are, of course, nothing new. Recently, however, a number of films have focused on the themes of sexually transmitted plagues, corrosive body fluids, or the fatal consequences of extramarital sex.

Edward Guerrero (1990) comments on the frequent pessimistic endings in recent science-fiction and horror films: 'All seem to mediate a general feeling, permeating all areas of the social imagination and cultural production, of pessimism and disaster confronting a terminally-ill society' (Guerrero, 1990). He argues that two Hollywood sci-fi remakes, *The Thing* (1982) and *The Fly* (1986), and a British film, *Life Force* (1985), feature themes and imagery that excite and exploit the public dread of AIDS.

The Thing

The Thing Guerrero postulates as an 'allegory for the spread of AIDS through society.' No longer the humanoid vegetable of the 1950s original, the 1982 Thing is a powerful xenomorph, an alien being capable of invading, absorbing, and imitating humans and animals. Guerrero suggests that 'much of the xenomorph's power to frighten its audience . . . is due to the close analogy between the Thing's behavior and what was known of the epidemiological behavior of the agent causing the "gay plague." ' The monster's *modus operandi* clearly parallels the virus's geometric spread due to its long period of asymptomatic latency, and the driving terror behind most of the film's action is that of not knowing who has been penetrated and replicated by the Thing. Moreover, the sociological setting of the action suggests it was intended to parody the homosexual enclaves most vulnerable to the epidemic. The location is a station in Antarctica, a 'bi-racial, isolated homosocial world in which . . . the crew overindulge in alcohol and open pot smoking.' Guerrero observes that in 1982, 'AIDS was generally looked upon as a disease afflicting an isolated world of homosexuals; marginal men who were, because of their indulgent lifestyles, responsible for their own pollution.'

In the context of this microcosmic representation of a gay world, Guerrero notes, the climactic scene possesses a certain metaphorical power. The protagonist decides to subject the remaining members of the crew to a blood test by drawing a hot wire through a

Petri dish, with dramatic results: '. . . xeno-contaminated blood leaps from the dish and flows towards its parent Thing, which erupts out of the blood- soaked human shell in which it has been dissembling.' This scene conveys the social reality of a positive HIV test: 'the exploding metaphor of the monster unmasked.' It is significant, as Guerrero points out, that the scene emphasizes 'both the wilful mobility of the contaminated blood, as well as the extravagant splatterings of gelatinous, bloody slime,' for the effect of this is 'to play upon the irrational fear building in the public imagination of contaminated body fluids and blood imbued with conscious intent, ready to leap out and infect America's middle-class majority under conditions of the most casual contact.'

The Fly

In *The Fly* (1986) the concern is not with the progress of an epidemic, but rather with the 'the slow, agonizing deterioration of its protagonist's body.' As in the 1958 version, the plot originates in the accidental mixing of fly and human genes, leading to the slow destruction of a brilliant scientist. Unlike the married man of the earlier version, the protagonist (Jeff Goldblum) is single, and the film is an 'exploration of the upscale, singles' sexual liberation and . . . its dreaded pathological consequences, all of which draws upon public alarm over new sexually transmitted diseases emergent in the 1980s.' The scientist's 'geometrically increasing sexual appetite as his accidentally transplanted fly genes activate' and the film's 'numerous explicit lovemaking scenes' conspire to evoke 'public suspicion of promiscuous sexual activity as one of the causes of AIDS.' To drive the point home, the protagonist, reacting to the mutation of his decaying body, phones his girlfriend to warn her that he's 'got something,' a 'bizarre form of cancer' and 'it might be contagious.'

Guerrero does not comment on the most horrific scene of all, when the protagonist, at an advanced stage of metamorphosis, spews corrosive saliva over his girlfriend's persistent ex-lover's leg, reducing it to a charred stump of bone. The message here appears to be that, in a lovers' triangle, body fluids can be lethal.

In another scene of possible significance the mutant scientist tries to convince his pregnant girlfriend to enter his machine, the 'pod,' in order to mix their genes and dilute the fly component and emerge as one human being: 'We'll be the ultimate family,' he coaxes her. This could be interpreted as an ironic comment on the deformation of the modern family and its vulnerability to the con-tamination of AIDS.

Life Force

The third film, *Life Force* (1985), Guerrero sees as 'negotiating so-cietal dread of both the etiological and the epidemiological mani-festations of the [AIDS] syndrome.' *Life Force* is set in London and portrays a society ravished by a pandemic caused by a 'vampiristic xenomorphic form' from outer space which, on planet earth, chooses to replicate itself as a beautiful, naked young woman. The sexually alluring xenomorph infects the population through a deadly kiss which sucks the 'life force' out of its victims, leaving behind a string of desiccated corpses who rise up as vampires to feed on the life force of others, 'thus spreading the contamination geometrically and giving the film its distinctly epidemiological character' (Guerrero, 1990:92).

The implied moral of these films is a conservative one. Guerrero notes, 'although *The Thing* argues the threat of AIDS to homosex-uals and *The Fly* threatens heterosexuals . . . both films implicitly ratify the safety and sanctity of the monogamous "traditional" family.' A similar message is conveyed in the final scene of *Life Force*, in which the hero plunges a sword through the embracing bodies of himself and the xenomorph, thereby liberating the life force of thousands of human souls about to be siphoned up in a glowing column into the hatch of a hovering alien starship. Guer-rero comments:

> The aggrandized, paradigmatic image of a naked heterosexual union centered in the *mise en scène* of a cathedral subtly, implicitly argues that the dominant ideology of romance, marriage, and heterosexu-

ality has more than a little to do with the plague's cessation and containment.

After reading Guerrero's article, one begins to see hidden references to AIDS in any film that deals with destructive sex or disgusting body fluids, from *Alien* to *Little Shop of Horrors*. Two recent films, however, *Fatal Attraction* and *Project Alien*, dramatize the ambivalent attitudes towards premarital and extramarital sex found in our society, an ambivalence that the advent of AIDS has highlighted. Both films celebrate the glamour of what Mormon leaders would term 'sexual adventurism' and, at the same time, warn us of its life-threatening consequences.

Fatal Attraction

Fatal Attraction (1988) reflects the conflicting views in our culture towards adultery, and warns against the psychological and physical dangers resulting from a casual, short-lived love affair. The protagonist (Michael Douglas) meets an attractive, sophisticated professional (Glenn Close) who, in the course of the action, is transformed into a raging, psychopathic harpy wreaking vengeance on his marriage, children, house, and reputation. Douglas appears as a kind, eminently reasonable, but 'averagely adulterous' man who is struggling to maintain a firm barrier between a weekend of spontaneous lust and his disciplined daily life as a professional and family man. He desperately appeals to the original contract struck with his lover in embarking on their weekend fling and, in a final 'gender battle,' resorts to killing the she-monster in self-defence.

The gender-war dénouement appears to be one of the 1980s' most startling innovations. Further examples include *Jagged Edge*, in which Glenn Close shoots her lover when he turns out to be the evil murderer. In another film, *Misery* (1990), a pulp writer is held captive by a fan and escapes her preparations for a romantic double suicide by killing her.

As *Fatal Attraction* appeared in 1988, at the peak of the AIDS scare, it could be argued that it conforms to Guerrero's theory and is an allegory or cautionary tale about the threat that AIDS poses to one's social identity and to the family unit. Glenn Close, in the final struggle, her blond hair wild, a loose, cream-coloured dress stretched across her swollen belly, could be the virus personified, attacking the head of the family in his own bathroom. The film's explicit love-making scenes take place in rickety, rising elevators, or against the banisters of steep staircases, suggesting a sudden fall or public exposure. The final message is that a brief sexual liaison, thought to be buried in the past, can suddenly rear up as a monster and attack one's reputation and loved ones.

Project Alien

Project Alien (1990), a Frank Shields film, starts out as an alien invasion story when a reporter is sent to investigate a possible UFO sighting in connection with a missing plane. In order to reconnoitre the Norwegian forest, he hires a pilot who turns out to be a woman; a beautiful nymphomaniac, a reckless driver, and a flamboyant aviatrix. Together they find evidence of a mysterious wasting plague that leaves cancerous sores on its victims. Suspecting extra-terrestrial weapons, they eventually realize that the disease is the accidental by-product of military experiments in biological warfare. They stumble upon a secret hospital where the victims of the plague are imprisoned and subjected to experimental cures in a cover-up operation involving the Soviet and U.S. governments. Throughout the investigation, the reporter (Mike Nouri) resists the aviatrix's sexual advances. His self-control is dramatized by his habit of holding an unlit cigarette in his fingers until he finally feels like breaking it – while she smokes uninhibitedly. In the final scene, after the cause of the mysterious plague has been deter-mined, he jumps into bed with her. The plot suggests a nostalgic return to the sexual revolution after the 'plague' is de-mystified and contained. It also resonates with conspiracy theories pointing to political motives behind the origin and spread of AIDS.

Poison

Todd Haynes's *Poison* (1991), unlike the more commercial films cited above, is self-consciously metaphorical in its references to AIDS. Asked in an interview whether he intended to make a 'specific parable about AIDS, ' the filmmaker replied:

> I was very conscious of 'AIDS' as a metaphor. The same way that Genet as a writer and thinker influences the film as a whole, similarly the shadow cast by 'AIDS' affects the whole film as well, even though the Horror section is more explicitly related to it. There, clearly, a diseased person is considered a threat to society. (Satuloff, 1991:11)

Haynes explains in the same interview that the idea behind *Poison* was to have 'three stories that weren't necessarily related, set in different periods, with different characters. By intercutting the three, I thought it would get the audience to think about the larger issues underneath each story.'

These three tales of transgression and punishment, titled *Hero*, *Horror*, and *Homo*, belong to different genres. *Horror* is a black-and-white 1950s monster movie in which the protagonist, Dr Graves, accidentally drinks the sex-drive essence potion that he has isolated and transforms into the 'Leper Sex-Killer,' a hideously pustular monster who pounds the pavements after dark, transmitting instant leprosy to subservient blond women. *Hero* is a mock-documentary shot in colour in which a Long Island housewife is interviewed in her kitchen and relates how her seven-year-old son, Richie, shot his wife-battering, child-beating father dead and then jumped out a second-storey window and flew up to heaven. *Homo* is a Genet-influenced romantic study of the life of Broom, a child falsely accused of stealing, who spends a bucolic boyhood in Borstal and in manhood discovers the mystical dimensions of homosexual love and brutality in prison. What unites the film is the theme of bodily fluids, which binds the film in an intricate web of cross-references. Dr Graves's leprous running sores are visually rhymed in the *Homo* sequence in which a teenage boy is ritualistically spat upon by his schoolmates, his mouth held open in a silent cry of anguish as rose petals and phlegm rain from the heavens in a cascade of humiliation – and in a parody of Christian martyrdom. *Hero* echoes the theme of disgusting body effluvia employed in making statements about social hierarchy when a Long Island neighbour relates in an interview how the mysteriously vanished boy-angel once leaped over her fence into her garden, naked 'like a wild animal,' and deliberately defecated on her lawn.

While Todd Haynes defends the subtlety of his metaphor ('For people who need to figure things out and know exactly why things are occurring, *Poison* would be a very frustrating film. [It] doesn't have a single answer or message that it's trying to put out'), the film does imply a few judgments on hetero- versus homosexual relationships, and on power and pollution. It is significant that the 'kissing leprosy' afflicts heterosexuals, and a caricatured 1950s-style couple at that, in an era when American sex roles were at their most rigid. There is grim humour in the scenes when Real Woman-style Dr Olsen declares her love and dotes on her man, unaware that he is the Leper Sex-Killer. The message inferred could almost be that AIDS was generated out of the disembodied scientific curiosity and *hubris* of the all-male heterosexual society with its cloying ideals of romantic love. This sick society has created the homosexual and bequeathed its own brand of leprosy, created in a laboratory, to its monstrous child. All three stories are about how violent and brutal societies need to isolate and 'otherize' their abused children and to establish caste systems based on levels of pollution and purity.

AIDS: From Anomaly to Anomie

Many studies of society and AIDS have focused on the fear of the other, the anomalous, a fear often directed towards sexual, religious, and racial minorities. Stephen Schecter in his *AIDS Notebooks* (1990) traces society's homophobia to the terror of vagabonds throughout European history as carriers of pestilence, libertinism, heresy, and subversion. The vagabonds of the fourteenth century were rural immigrants and 'déclassé rejects of a declining feudal order.' The sixteenth and seventeenth centuries added disbanded regiments of soldiers who turned to brigandage. The chiliastic, egalitarian movements of European history which Norman Cohn (1970) and Kenelm Burridge (1969) have explained as 'protorevolutionary movements' or 'religions of the dispossessed' attracted large numbers of vagabonds and those who escaped martyrdom 'provided the revolutionary incendiarism for the revolts that shook the *ancien régime*.' By the nineteenth century, Schecter argues, the vagabond had become the utopian who resisted the ascendancy of bourgeois society. His wandering was effectively curtailed by the creation of poorhouses, hospitals, schools, prisons, and other examples of 'institutional reform ... that typify bourgeois rationality.' Schecter then raises the question of who today's vagabonds are, and suggests that, besides beatniks, hippies, political refugees, and colonial immigrants, it is homosexuals: 'they, too, [cross] boundaries in the geography of the body and even more so in the fantasy world that structures it.'

In the movies and other popular media, stories about people with AIDS proliferate: some of them monstrous and others endearingly human. There are people who overcome their own disabilities to help others, and there are people who transmit the disease to others unconsciously or intentionally; some die from it and others refuse to die. These stories awaken our anxieties and then allay them by defining – and redefining – what is truly human or 'normal.' An outrageous PWA such as Michael Callen has crossed the boundaries of what is generally considered human, healthy, ethical. He boasts of receiving '3,000 people up my ass' and has caught 'every STD in the book several times.' Even so, he has managed to come back home, a prodigal son, to live on for a decade and to tell his tale, and this helps his listeners redefine the limits of normalcy, of health, and of 'human-ness.' Perhaps, after hearing his story, some of his listeners will never look on those boundaries as quite so inflexible and insurmountable.

Goldstein (1987) has observed that AIDS just so happens to combine certain characteristics that 'have the capacity to reinvigorate ancient stereotypes' AIDS is remarkable because it is 'the first epidemic to take stigmatized classes and make them victims.'

What are these 'ancient stereotypes' that are 'reinvigorated' by

PWA stories and recent movies that contain horrifying images of xenomorphs, vampires, and the living dead?

Psychohistorical insights into monsters are offered in Leslie Fiedler's *Freaks* (1978), which explores some of the fantasies surrounding anomalous births, non-white races, and hermaphrodites in European Christendom. Fiedler notes that in early Christian communities deformed babies evoked a sense of religious awe as signs of God's wrath, or as omens or portents. The fascination and folklore concerning freaks, he argues, is an expression of 'our psychological need to create monsters' to deal with 'our basic uncertainty about the limits of our bodies and our egos.' This uncertainty is rooted in children's experience of growing up; their changing height, the growth of pubic hair – 'more like animal fur than that on their heads' – and the swelling parts of their bodies in puberty. He describes the sexuality of the pre-pubescent child as 'bisexual, polymorphous, perverse'; constantly 'aggravated by the adult world's changing views of their sexual viability.' The sex freaks popular in the nineteenth century were the 'incarnate symbols of the [Victorian child's] distress . . . the Eunuch, the girl without a vulva, the Hottentot Venus with labia halfway down to her thighs, and especially the Hermaphrodite: Joseph-Josephine, Half Man/ Half Woman' (Fiedler, 1978:39). He claims, moreover, that regardless of the sexual codes of the surrounding culture, 'the child is bound to feel some monstrous discrepancy between his erotic nature and the role expectations of his era.'

I would argue that some of the media's portraits of PWAs and the reports of racial and sexual minorities as conduits for the 'new plague' provide a similar function to that of Victorian freak shows. They seem to awaken primordial fears regarding our sexuality, our tenuous individuality, and our status as more than beasts. PWAs and racist stereotypes – like Fiedler's 'true freak' – challenge the 'conventional boundaries between male and female, sexed and sexless, animal and human . . . self and other, and consequently between reality and illusion, experience and fantasy, fact and myth' (Fiedler, 1978:40).

EIGHT

AIDS, Symbols, and Society

AIDS and the Nation, AIDS and the Family, AIDS and the Individual,
AIDS and the American Way of Death,
The Future: Apocalypse or Accommodation?

Susan Sontag (1989) has evoked the mood of helpless pessimism marking the close of the twentieth century in her epigram describing the generational shift from a political paranoia in the 1950s to an exospheric-paranoia in the 1980s. 'Apocalypse,' she states, 'has become a long-running serial, not 'Apocalypse Now,' but 'Apocalypse from Now On.'

This might describe the march of AIDS by the end of the second millennium CE. When we, the denizens of the late twentieth century, look back from our self-righteously scientific perspective on the bubonic plague, we are appalled by the panic-driven behaviour of church and town. People carried pomanders filled with aromatic spices to ward off the putatively infectious miasmas wafting through the air. Medieval physicians lacked our diagnostic methods to locate the true source of the buboes – flea-infested rats. Hence, their rigid quarantines and scapegoatings were stringently enforced but completely useless. Today, everyone understands how AIDS is spread through blood and semen – and yet our fragmented, pluralistic society lacks the impressive social control of a medieval village and is incapable of protecting its members. In 1983 the word 'epidemic' was cautiously applied – inside quotations. Today, 'pandemic' is the term almost routinely used – and quotation marks have been discarded. In 1983 the numbers were low, and the AIDS virus might have been erased from the planet if draconian measures of testing and quarantine had been rigorously enforced. We may expect far more serious infringements of human rights and privacy if the public health system collapses beneath the weight of world victims. In this situation, people will turn to religion, 'one of the most effective bulwarks against anomie' (Berger, 1969:87). And in the midst of this urgency, apocalyptic religions will appear increasingly relevant.

If proof be needed that external events in the world situation have conspired to fuel ancient apocalyptic myths, one need only look at an organization in San Francisco called Doom, the Society for Secular Armageddonism. A toll-free telephone call will enable concerned citizens to hear the following recorded message:

> We believe the apocalypse is at hand, and the reasons for that belief are overwhelming: chemical and biological weapons, nuclear proliferation, deforestation, the greenhouse effect, ozone depletion, acid rain, the poisoning of our air and water, rising racism, massive species loss, toxic waste, the AIDS pandemic, the continuing population explosion, encroaching Big Brotherism, and at least a thousand points of blight . . . and they're all proof that we don't need God to do it for us. The coming end will be a strictly do-it-yourself apocalypse. (*Harper's Magazine*, December 1990)

A similar mood of awful dread is conveyed throughout the media's coverage of the AIDS crisis. While news reports might focus on scientific and statistical findings, their carefully rational tone is belied by hysterical headlines thundering apocalyptic messages across the front pages: 'SPEAKING OF THE PLAGUE!' screams *U.S. News & World Report* (17 June 1991); ET 'MASS KILLER SET TO BREAK OUT!' warns the *European* (5–7 July 1991). 'AIDS PANDEMIC, GLOBAL SCOURGE' bellows *Great Decisions* (1992). Headlines using biblical terms such as 'leper,' 'plague,' 'curse,' or 'scourge' cannot fail to invoke primordial fears. Titles such as 'The Advent of the HIV Virus' or 'The Coming of AIDS' (*American Spectator*, March 1986) ring millennial bells in the public's mind, and eloquently convey the epic scale of AIDS's expanding horrors. Other headlines appear almost to celebrate mass hysteria and sensationalize collective panic ('Virus of Fear,' *Houston Chronicle*, 15 September 1985; 'AIDS: At the Dawn of Fear,' *U.S. News & World Report*, 12 January 1987).

We find articles that self-consciously adopt religious themes, such as those that describe AIDS as an 'inferno,' the final *huis clos* of the damned. 'Doing Time in a Leper Colony' by Martin Delgado, *European*, and 'AIDS behind Bars' convey visions of the dark eschatologies forming in prisons. 'Inside an AIDS Colony' begins with a quote from Dostoevsky: 'Here was our own world, unlike anything else. Here were our own laws, our own dress . . . here was the house of the living dead.'

The psychohistorian Norman Cohn (1970), in his classic study of medieval millenarian movements, aroused some controversy among academics when he argued that contemporary Marxism bears all the major earmarks of ancient apocalyptic fantasies, albeit in secular guise. In a similar vein, a wealth of examples can be discovered in the popular press of the irresistible impulse to wax apocalyptic when confronted by a mysterious, fatal, and stigmatizing disease. The most striking example of secular AIDS-apocalypticism is perhaps an essay by John Platt (1987), 'The Future of AIDS.'

Calling AIDS 'the Black Death in slow motion,' Platt predicts it could 'wipe out some countries' and 'delayed deaths could even begin to cancel out our rapid world population growth.' By the year 2000, 'there will be new behaviours, new social structures, and new global relations in a world that even five years ago we could not have imagined.' His dark vision resembled science fiction in 1987, but today it is not implausible:

> Our social behaviour . . . will become increasingly remniscent of life during earlier plagues. Hospitals will become desperately overcrowded, and many will die at home or be abandoned. Burials will be replaced by cremations . . . hopelessness . . . will alternate with an 'eat drink and be merry' philosophy. Victims of AIDS will grow violent, furious with this world . . . [Many] will commit suicide to avoid months of suffering and enormous cost to their families. There would likely be more legal and religious approval of euthanasia . . . Food might be bought and served only in sealed packets . . . people may avoid public toilets, restaurants, crowds and even public transportation. Work, play, education would be concentrated in the 'elec-

tronic cottage' with the main connection to the outside being through the networks of a video universe. (Platt, 1987:15–16)

There are, of course, countless articles on AIDS that eschew metaphors and simply report the facts. But no matter how scrupulously restrained and scientific the tone of the writing may be, if the iconography and illustrations chosen to embellish them depict the Grim Reaper or dancing skeletons from medieval or Reformation woodcuts, these threaten the reader with the image of Death personified.

Thus AIDS has become a witty and palpable symbol in the secular sphere, where vague and formless feelings of threat can find a focus. These deeply felt threats to identity seem to exist on four levels: the planetary, the national, the familial, and the individual.

AIDS and the Nation

Loss of certainty at the national level is expressed in conspiracy theories concerning the dissemination of AIDS, or in critiques of the way the epidemic has been handled by politicians, doctors, and public health officials. Thus far, gay groups, the LaRouchians, the Rajneesh, and the Church Universal and Triumphant have been the most vociferous in their complaints. AIDS might be the final blow to American 'civil religion,' first described by de Tocqueville, and reaching its peak in the Jacksonian brand of optimistic postmillennialism. The fearful prospect of America being subverted and dominated by an outside, proselytizing, hostile, global communism (an image that gripped the social imagination in the 1950s) appears to have been replaced by an uneasiness regarding what Douglas would call 'pollution from within.' The dread of communist subversion of the body politic in the 1950s has shifted to a 1990s paranoia concerning the pandemic spread of bacterial, viral, and chemical pollutants through our physical bodies. Media stories have appeared that express this notion – that the corruption is already deeply imbedded within our society ('The Plague Within,' *Equinox*, November/December 1987, and 'AIDS and Panic: Enemies Within,' *Wall Street Journal*, 28 April 1987), whereas others focus xenophobically on external invaders ('AIDS: Fear of Foreigners,' *Newsweek*, 6 April 1987; 'AIDS at Our Door: Preparing for an Unwanted Guest,' *Corrections Today*, February 1990).

The post-Nixonian disillusionment with authority figures permeates AIDS media stories, targeting doctors, dentists, and other health professionals, as conveyed in such stories as 'Physicians with AIDS' (*St Louis Post Dispatch*, 19 May 1991), or 'Should You Worry about Getting AIDS from Your Dentist?' (*Time*, 29 July 1991) or 'Nurse with AIDS Tells Her Story' (Ft Lauderdale *Sun Sentinel*, 27 September 1990).

AIDS can be used to justify or deplore the process of globalization. As Susan Sontag points out, 'the AIDS crisis is evidence of a world in which nothing important is regional, local, limited; in which every problem is . . . worldwide.' She foresees national integrity, cultural identity – and the taboos that protect them – fast becoming obsolete:

> People circulate, in greater numbers than ever. And diseases. From the untrammeled intercontinental air travel . . . to the unprecedented migrations of the underprivileged . . . all this physical mobility and inter-connectedness (with its consequent dissolving of old taboos, social and sexual) is . . . vital to the maximum functioning of the advanced, or world, capitalist economy . . . (Sontag, 1989:92)

John Platt (1987:12) argues that AIDS may transform international politics, uniting major powers in a 'life-and-death interest that laughs at the nation-state.' Optimistically, he suggests that a 'new New Deal will be called for . . . paid for by cancelling other expensive projects – big science, fusion power, space stations, the Strategic Defense Initiative – that will seem increasingly irrelevant in a world dominated by AIDS.' He optimistically predicts, 'The challenge of coping with AIDS at all levels could give the world a new sense of planet-wide interdependence and responsibility for human survival.'

AIDS and the Family

AIDS metaphors can also refer to the threatened integrity of the American nuclear family and the shifting boundaries between male and female. Lawrence Stone (1977) and Mary Ann Glendon (1985) have identified and analysed some of the dramatic changes in the patterns of family life and in the roles of women in the industrialized societies of North America and Western Europe. They point to the impact of cultural movements such as women's liberation, the gay movement, the sexual revolution, birth control, and the quest for individual autonomy on the modern family. These changes have taken an emotional toll on individuals, and have created considerable confusion concerning the basic rules governing interpersonal relationships and sexual identity.

AIDS stories reflect these tensions, and often dramatize the ambiguity surrounding gender issues in today's society. News reports express a lack of trust between men and women ('When He Has AIDS – And She Doesn't Know,' *American Health*, January/February 1991). The perils of male-female relations are underscored, as in the following AIDS stories: 'Heterosexuals and AIDS: Loving Dangerously' (Ft Lauderdale *Sun Sentinel*, 10 November 1991); 'AIDS and Heterosexuals: Worry But Don't Worry' (*News and Views*, January/February 1987); 'The Big Chill . . . How Heterosexuals Are Coping with a Disease That Can Make Sex Deadly,' (*Time*, 16 February 1987).

There are vampire/harpy stories of vengeful, dangerous female AIDS carriers, such as the beautiful black woman who picked up men in Miami bars to avenge herself on the male sex: 'Tale of Revenge Stirs AIDS Furor: Woman Claims She's Trying to Infect Men, Prompting a Surge of Concern' (*The New York Times*, 18 October 1991:A16). Recently, from Edmonton, Canada, a beautiful Filipina ex-model hit the headlines in a 'hell hath no fury' tale. She was charged with deliberately injecting her photographer-lover with HIV-infected blood during two of their sadomasochistic sex episodes (*The Globe and Mail*, 10 May 1995).

Considering our culture's conflicting messages regarding gender roles and the growing intolerance for bisexuality in the main-

stream, it might be argued that today's condom ads express concerns above and beyond pure hygiene. As Douglas (1966:122)
observes, in societies where 'some of the basic postulates are denied
by other basic postulates, so that the system seems to be at war
with itself,' the body-as-symbol is used in a kind of 'unfunny wit'
to express danger to community boundaries. Douglas explains this
as follows:

> Both male and female physiology lend themselves to the analogy
> with the vessel which must not pour away or dilute its vital fluids.
> Females are correctly seen as literally the entry by which the pure
> fluid may be adulterated. Males are treated as pores through which
> the precious stuff may ooze out and be lost, the whole system thereby
> enfeebled.

Gays transgressing the boundaries separating male from female,
therefore, are perceived as anomalous, with bodies that combine
the imperfect container with the leaky sponge. If they also happen
to carry a contagious disease transmitted through bodily fluids,
they become powerful symbols of social disorder – especially for
small, threatened societies. Considering that the contemporary
Western family is rapidly mutating and gender roles are 'up for
grabs,' it is hardly surprising that notions of sexual pollution are
flourishing in post-industrial societies today. The urban dweller's
fear of AIDS appears to fulfil a similar social function to pollution
fears in primitive tribes (Douglas, 1966:141). It is 'enlisted to bind
men and women to their allotted roles.'

AIDS and the Individual

I am utterly convinced, after watching the xenomorph explode in
the 1982 movie *The Thing*, that AIDS provides an apt metaphor for
the loss of our social identity or 'face,' and for the real and imagined
daily assaults on our human integrity. For the individual, the fear
of AIDS involves a reluctance to go through what the poor protagonist suffers in the 1986 remake of *The Fly* – a hideous, embarrassing, and literal 'loss of face' (parts of his face fall off in the course

of his metamorphosis). Goffman (1968:5) defines 'face' as 'an image of self delineation in terms of approved social attributes,' 'a social construction that people depend on others to support.' Those who fail to support other peoples' 'face' will be perceived as dangerous, and people who take on roles they cannot sustain are 'out of face,' thereby posing a threat to others – who are then obliged to witness their embarrassing 'loss of face.' News stories concerning PWAs who conceal their HIV status from lovers or co-workers, as in 'Faces of an Epidemic' (*Washington Post*, 10 February 1997:6) or 'To Know or Not to Know?' (*American Health*, September 1987) express much more than simply the fear of disease. The story 'To Test or Not to Test' (Collins, 1987) quotes people's trepidations concerning AIDS tests and the possible consequence of facelessness: 'It's another nightmare I just don't need in this crazy country,' says one woman. 'I'd be really terrified if I tested positive.' 'No, I just don't have to think about it,' says another. Even among those who undergo testing, there are 'people who won't pick up their test results because they can't handle it emotionally.'

This fear of facelessness in a fluid world, where personal commitments are increasingly transient and social boundaries are constantly shifting, seems to have found a focus in AIDS. The unique combination of the virus's features make it a convenient symbol for the complex and paradoxical sense of pollution and danger people feel in a society that demands they juggle a range of roles simultaneously, while the relationships they depend on to maintain their sacred sense of self have become increasingly fragmented.

AIDS and the American Way of Death

The advent of AIDS has had a profound effect upon the way Americans view death. In a society where, until recently, death was a 'forbidden subject' (Gorer, 1965), excluded from conversation and purged from public awareness, the exponential spread of a disease that is utterly mysterious, stigmatizing, and fatal reminds us of the reality and terrible finality of death.

Geoffrey Gorer has observed that death fills a niche in modern society that is not dissimilar to the place of sex in the Victorian age, and he argues that death, now secret and forbidden, has become 'the new pornography.' Chidester (1990:260) traces the modern tendency to 'medicalize' death back to the nineteenth century, when scientific naturalism gradually emerged to dominate American attitudes towards death and dying. Unseen causes of death could now be revealed through a microscope and fought through medical procedures. Even old age was included in science's war on death. Nobel laureate Ellie Metchnikoff expressed an extreme version of this attitude when he diagnosed old age as 'an infectious disease' and promised optimistically that 'it should be possible to cure it or postpone it' (Aries, 1981:587).

The advent of AIDS undermines the prevailing 'American way of death' and restores our lost sense of terror and mystery. Thus far, the HIV virus has eluded scientists, for its shape keeps changing and a cure has not been found. It is defined in negative terms – as a failure of the immune system to protect the body from 'opportunistic diseases' – almost as if the affliction were an absence of health rather than the presence of disease. Media stories concerning the refusal of individual doctors, nurses, and public health officials to accept PWAs as their clients dramatize the triumph of primitive fear or superstition over the rational competence expected of these professionals. Shrouded in mystery, AIDS poses a serious challenge to the 'medicalization of death.'

By the mid-1980s, the public's growing awareness and horror of the magnitude of the danger and the future toll of this new disease seemed to augur a resurgence of the 'savage death' that elicits a fascination with the macabre. In trying to ignore death, Aries (1981) argues, we only increase our fear of evil, for it is no longer recognized as a part of human nature, but is banished to marginal areas – war, crime, racism, incest. Since he finds the belief in evil essential for the taming of death, 'the disappearance of the belief has restored death to its savage state' (Aries, 1981:613).

The skeleton of medieval rhetoric has been replaced by the popular image of the macabre – the dying hospital patient, covered with tubes – the hideous mask of medical technology. With the decline of the romantic era and the 'beautiful death,' illness and pain arouse not pity, but distaste. We belong, Aries argues, to the era of the 'invisible death,' when death becomes 'dirty and medicalized,' gradually more and more surreptitious, violent, and savage. Death by AIDS arouses the same strange curiosity, the same 'perverse deviations and eroticism' as a tale by Edgar Allan Poe. The 'living dead' stories of beautiful PWAs who vengefully contaminate, the myth of the erection of the hanged man, and the fear of premature entombment – all express the same preoccupation with that 'impure and reversible state that partakes of both life and death' (Aries, 1982:608–9), inspiring emotions mingling desire and fear.

A striking example of this is 'Love Stories in the Age of AIDS' (Schoofs, 1994), which relates four case histories of 'sero-discordant' or 'magnetic' couples – where one partner is dying but the other somehow remains HIV negative. The narrative tone is romantic, offering 'travellers' tales' of 'mixed couples who live and love in a psychological territory that remains largely uncharted.'

AIDS is strangely, erotically compelling in these narratives. The protagonists reveal a fatalistic fascination with risky sex and observe an esoteric etiquette that considers it selfishly unromantic to avoid sexual relationships with HIV-positive men – or even, in the event of overpowering attraction to a PWA, to wear a condom. To flirt with death constitutes a deep emotional surrender and an added sexual stimulation:

> After the death of his lover to AIDS, Scott was on the verge of making a decision which, even now, I dread. 'I want my next lover to be HIV negative and I have considered ruling out all positives.' 'That's not politically correct!' his (HIV-positive) therapist told him. He concludes 'I haven't adopted a no-positives policy, partly because it feels like slapping [his deceased lover] in the face. Then, too, it's generally believed that half the gay men in this city are infected with HIV, so I cringe at ruling out so many men. Finally, there's desire . . . he was smart, sexy, full of fun . . . by resolving only to hope [my next lover is HIV negative] I am letting my unconscious in its impenetrable tangle of guilt and horror and desire, make this decision for me.'

These testimonials of gays in love with the dying are existential rebellions against death: 'I think the length of time somebody lives is beside the point.' They are new formulations of that ancient cry: *finis vitae sed non amoris* ('It is the end of life but not of love'). But they also possess a macabre edge:

> Greg believes he possesses a 'toxic cock' and is tormented by the possibility that he infected the great love of his life, Ray, who died in 1989. In nightmares he is haunted by the faces of ghosts . . . men he has loved and, he fears, slain.
>
> .   .   .
>
> Alex is necking with his new friend but remembers his deceased lover, so that images of suffering become superimposed on the present . . . 'It was now David's blood in the mixing bowl, David's skin, yellow against the hospital sheets and gray against the sheets in the morgue. My erection slumped.'

In its early phases, AIDS was neither beautiful nor natural in the popular imagination. It was associated with 'unnatural' acts and with artificial origins. In stark contrast with romantic views of death, such as 'Mother Nature's soft bosom' (Chidester, 1990:258), AIDS was explained as 'nature's backlash' – the consequence of meddling with or abusing nature (e.g., preservatives in food, pollutants in the environment). More recent portraits of dying PWAs, however, suggest that we might be witnessing a return to the 'romantic way of death.' In the daytime soaps beautiful PWAs kiss and marry millionaires. Extravagant balls and fund-raising benefits presided over by legendary film stars such as Elizabeth Taylor lend a glamour to the disease and endow the afflicted with a sense of dignity. Famous artists and actors such as Rudolf Nureyev and Anthony Perkins die surrounded by luxury and loving friends. Their last statements, words of insight and altruism, are reverently quoted. These scenes suggest a revival of the *artes moriendi*, the public, ritualized deathbed scene. Ma Jaya, Florida high priestess of the art of dying with dignity, is in the vanguard of this movement.

As death by AIDS grows more familiar – and hence more tame – there are efforts made to beautify it. As we move into the mid-1990s we begin to find many examples of the 'romantic way of death' among artistic expressions of grief and emotion by friends, lovers, and family members of dying PWAs. These works shift attention away from the patient or the deceased to the survivors' feelings of loss.

The Future: Apocalypse or Accommodation

If – or perhaps I should say when – a cure for AIDS is found, the statements recorded above will become no more than curiosities. If, however, the virus continues to spread exponentially and reach pandemic proportions, the possible repercussions for religion include the following:

- *The renewal of religion's function of preserving the sanctity of the family.* The AIDS threat will continue to be used to reinforce individual churches' particular versions of sexuality and family life, and to prove that these are divinely ordained or reflect a higher order.

- *A resurgence of millenarian movements.* The advent of AIDS as we approach the year 2000 has evidently stimulated the apocalyptic fantasies of minority churches, and this is likely to increase as we advance towards the second millennium. The old religious idioms have been replaced by secular ones, but, as Norman Cohn (1972:286) observes, 'it is the simple truth that, stripped of their original supernatural sanction, revolutionary millenarianism and mystical anarchism are with us still.'

- *The proliferation of healing cults.* Out of those churches which hold that illness reflects a state of sin or inferior consciousness, new healing mystiques and rituals are likely to arise – especially since Antiviral and other drugs permit PWAs to live longer. Therapeutic cults originating in the human potential movement and New Age groups are likely to respond in this fashion, while gay spiritual responses will probably recede as the virus claims more and more heterosexual victims.

As Christopher Evans noted in *Cults of Unreason* (1974), charismatic leaders have often displayed an almost uncanny ability to predict future trends. In 1984 Rajneesh began insisting on condoms and AIDS tests. By 1987 singles' clubs in New York were instituting obligatory HIV testing for their members. Unificationists incorporated this practice into their Blessings in 1986, and today many engaged couples in the mainstream are unwittingly following their example. Communal societies such as the Northeast Kingdom and The Family insist on AIDS tests for new members. Even the LaRouchians note self-righteously in their paper that 'AIDS reports 1991 sound like LaRouche 1984.'

Finally, if AIDS does continue to spread exponentially, and if increased pressure is placed on public health, legal, and political authorities to solve the problem, religion might turn out to offer the best protection for individuals and families. Religious communities are uniquely qualified to provide enclaves of safety owing to their ability to exert a stringent control over their members' courtship patterns and reproductive faculties. The famous historian of the family, Lawrence Stone, interviewed on Canadian television, was invited to extrapolate on the social consequences of a widespread epidemic, and postulated the following developments:

My guess is that a totalitarian state will emerge which will impose very, very severe restrictions on the victims and will also change sexual relationships, or drive people back into monogamous relationships – whether they like it or not!

It would appear likely that legal measures, public health rules, or even a totalitarian regime will fail to stem contagion or effectively segregate the infected. In the end, it will be those communities that can control the sexual behaviour of their youth that will be the least threatened by AIDS. These will include sects of established religions, such as the Hassidim, the Amish, and the Mormons, besides communal 'cults' such as the Moonies, Krishnas, and 3HOs, which have developed systems for supervising courtship and arranging marriages. Secular fortresses shutting out the surrounding plague will very likely emerge out of corporations, political parties, or health clubs, paralleling religious communes in their rules and ideologies.

The reaction of the public, already described as 'overblown' and 'hysterical,' will undoubtedly continue to wax in irrationality if the number of infections increases. For this reason, fundamentalist and minority churches, with their apocalyptic visions, their healing rituals, their sexual, dietary, and blood taboos, are evidently better equipped to handle the irrational death traumas, pollution fears, and guilt feelings evoked by AIDS than mere secular authorities. Owing to their peculiar creativity in providing nomic constructions in which disease becomes metaphor, they can offer their congregations an effective shield against the anomic terror of AIDS.

Notes

1. Ellwood (1973) distinguishes a 'cult' from a 'sect' in the following manner: a *cult* is a small, ephemeral group formed around a living (or recently deceased) charismatic leader, whose members strive for ecstatic experience or esoteric knowledge and espouse a set of beliefs that deviate from the normative Judeo-Christian tradition. A *sect* is a voluntary society beyond its second generation, and often originating in a schism; its beliefs are orthodox in relation to its parent church, but its practices are strict and its way of life uncompromising, which places it in a 'sectarian' position *vis-à-vix* the larger society.
2. Much of this information on the Rajneesh Foundation was collected between 1984 and 1986 when their meditation centre and restaurant were operating on my street. During this period, I attended five therapy groups with members of the commune and interviewed around thirty *sannyasins*.
3. These statements are extracted from Ma Jivan Mada's presentation at the *Religion and AIDS* symposium on 1 December 1990, which was organized by Dr Arvind Sharma and myself and held at the Presbyterian College of McGill University, Montreal.
4. Personal communication.
5. This statement was presented at the *Religion and AIDS* symposium.
6. Yadurani Dasi presented this statement at the *Religion and AIDS* symposium.
7. My description of the Messianic Communities is based on informal research and participation observer methods over five years of visits to the Community in Island Pond, which is located near my country house.
8. This account of The Family and their response to AIDS is based on my research into their childrearing methods and visits to their communal

homes in San Diego, Washington, DC, Boston, Rio de Janeiro, Dunton Basset in Gloucestershire, Newcastle, London (England), Rome (Italy), Montreal, and Toronto. This research was funded by the Social Sciences and the Humanities Research Council and the Society for the Scientific Study of Religion.

9. This information was supplied by Amy Siskind, who grew up in the Sullivanian commune and is currently completing her doctoral dissertation on the movement at New York University.

10. This information was gleaned from conversations with leaders in the Free Daist Communion in Toronto in 1992.

11. This information was supplied by Mukunda of the Kashi Ashram, but I met Ma Jaya Bhagavati at the Communal Societies Association meeting in New Harmony, Indiana, in October 1993 and experienced some interesting personal reactions to her presence. Initially I found her outrageously *kitsch* in her taste and extroverted in her manner, as I sat next to her at dinner surrounded by her black-garbed gay *chelas*, with her kohl-ringed eyes and leopard-printed scarves. One *chela* spoke of her love for rollerblading, and of their daily skating processions on her ashram rink. I watched her depart the next day, flinging *japas* around the neck of a new disciple, then settling into her Greyhound bus installed with kidney-shaped 1950s-style furniture upholstered in plastic leopard design. Somehow, it was hard to take her seriously. But after reading her long prose-poem, *The River*, and finding out more about her work with the dying, I began to wonder if she might not be one of the great saints of our century.

12. This account of the Raelians is based on eight years of intermittent research at their monthly meetings with my Dawson College students where, for educational purposes, we have been conducting membership surveys and interviewing members.

13. Personal communication.

14. Personal communication.

15. Personal communication.

16. This account of the Ansaars is partly based on long conversations with the disciples at their craft booths in Times Square, Manhattan, and at the Eaton Centre in Toronto. I also managed to collect interviews with two former members of the Montreal commune.

17. Information on the Aryan Nations was kindly supplied by James Aho, Michael Barkun, and Rob Balch. Aho wrote the brilliant *Politics of Righteousness* and sent me some of their literature. More of their (appalling) newsletters were supplied by a black friend who is on the Nations' subscription

list. Since I was worried about being investigated by the Royal Canadian Mounted Police, who were interviewing people in my area who had (involuntarily) been receiving Ku Klux Klan pamphlets in the mail, I asked him to collect material for me, since he had already been questioned by the puzzled RCMP and argued convincingly that he was not a white racist.

References

Adams, Moody. 1986. *AIDS: You Just Think You're Safe*. Baker, Los Angeles: Dalton Moody Publishers.

Aho, James A. 1990. *The Politics of Righteousness*. Seattle & London: University of Washington Press.

'AIDS: An Adventist Perspective.' 1986. *Adventist Review* (24 July 1986):1.

'The AIDS Conspiracy.' 1988. Livingston, MT: Summit University Forum (videocassette).

'AIDS a Global Killer: How Can You Protect Yourself?' 1988. *Awake!* (October). Watchtower Bible Society.

'AIDS: How to Protect Yourself: Will Science Find a Cure?' 1988. *The Plain Truth* (March).

'AIDS: Who Are at Risk?' 1986. *Awake!* (April).

'AIDS in the Workplace: A New Ruling Restricts Protection for Victims.' 1996. *Newsweek* (7 July):62.

Ammi, Ben. 1991. *The Messiah and the End of This World*. Washington, DC: Communicators Press.

'Are We in the Last Days?' 1988. *Awake!* (8 April):3.

Aries, Philippe. 1981. *The Hour of Our Death*. New York: Random House.

As Sayyid al Imaam Issa al Haadi al Mahdi. 1990. *The Paleman*. Brooklyn, NY: The Tents of Kedar.

'Back to the Garden: Death of a Snake Charmer.' 1992. *Freepaper*. Island Pond: VT.

Bamforth, Nick. 1987. *AIDS and the Healer Within*. New York: Amethyst Books.

Barker, Eileen. 1984. *The Making of a Moonie: Choice or Brainwashing?* Oxford: Blackwell.

Beckford, James. 1975. *The Trumpet of Prophecy*. Oxford: Basil Blackwell.

Bellah, Robert N. 1967. 'Civil Religion in America.' *Daedalus* 96 (1):1–21.

Bennett, Leslie. 1991. 'Marianne's Faithful.' *Vanity Fair* (June).

Benson, Ezra Taft. 1987. 'To the Home Teachers of the Church.' *Ensign Magazine* (May).

Berger, Peter. 1969. *The Sacred Canopy*. New York: Anchor Books.

Bhagavati, Ma Jaya Sati. 1994. 'At My Christ's Feet.' Sebastian, FL: Kashi Ashram.

Bhakti Abhay Charan Swami. 1990. 'AIDS and the Law of Karma.' Paper presented at the *Religion and AIDS* Symposium (1 April), McGill University, Montreal.

Bissinger, H.G. 1995. 'Lone Star Hate: On the Trail of Texas' Brutal Gay Killings.' *Vanity Fair* (February):80.

Bromley, David G. 1991. 'Satanism: The New Cult Scare.' *Society* 28 (May/June):55–66.

Bromley, David, & Philip Hammond, eds. 1987. *The Future of New Religious Movements*. Macon, GA: Mercer.

Brown, Norman. 1966. *Love's Body*. New York: Vintage Books.

Buck, Joan Juliet. 1992. 'Highlife and Lowlife.' *Vogue* (November):154.

Burridge, Kenelm. 1969. *New Heaven, New Earth: A Study of Millenarian Activities*. Oxford: Basil Blackwell.

Butterfield, Stephen. 1989. 'The Elephant in the Shrine Room.' *Shambala Sun*, Vol. 3 (Fall):17.

Cahalan, Kathleen A., ed. 1988. *AIDS: Issues in Religion, Ethics and Care*. Elmhurst, IL.: A Park Ridgeway Center Bibliography.

Callen, Michael. 1988. *Surviving and Thriving with Aids*. New York: People with AIDS Coalition.

Callwood, June. 1995. 'Date with AIDS.' *Saturday Night* (March):53.

Calvi, Giulia. 1984. *Histories of a Plague Year: The Social and the Imaginary in Baroque Florence*. Oxford: University of California Press.

Campbell, Colin. 1972. 'The Cult, the Cultic Milieu, and Secularization.' *A Sociological Yearbook of Religion in Britain* 5.

Carpenter, Edward. 1987. 'Selected Insights.' *Gay Spirit: Myth and Meaning*, edited by Mark Thompson. New York: St Martin's Press.

Carter, Lewis. 1987. 'The New Renunciates of Bhagwan Shree Rajneesh.' *Journal for the Scientific Study of Religion* 26(2):148–72.

Chidester, David. 1990. *Patterns of Transcendence*. Englewood Cliffs, NJ: Prentice-Hall.

'Children of Zaire: Victims of Secret AIDS Testing.' 1991. *Final Call* (5 August):9.

'Church and State Clash over AIDS Education.' *New York Times* (January 1988):B3.

Cohn, Norman. 1970. *The Pursuit of the Millennium*. London: Oxford University Press.

Conner, Daniel. 1987. 'Is AIDS the Answer to an Environmentalist's Prayer?' *Earth First!* (22 December):14–17.

Conrad, Peter. 1986. 'The Social Meaning of AIDS.' *Social Policy* 17(1):51–9.

A Course in Miracles. 1975. Chicago: The Foundation for Inner Peace.

de Courtivron, Isabelle. 1993. 'The Body Was His Battleground.' (Review of *The Passion of Michel Foucault* by James Miller.) *The New York Times Book Review* (10 January):1.

Davis-Barron, Sherri. 1992. 'Professor Sees AIDS as Punishing Homosexuals.' *Ottawa Citizen* (3 May):A9.

'Doctors Fear AIDS Too.' 1987. *Newsweek* (3 August):58.

Douglas, Mary. 1966. *Purity and Danger*. New York: Frederick Praeger.

Douglas, Mary. 1970. *Natural Symbols*. Harmondsworth: Penguin Books.

Dunne, Dominick. 1989. 'Robert Mapplethorpe's Long Goodbye.' *Vanity Fair* (February):124–33.

Durant, William, & Ariel Durant. 1968. *The Lessons of History*. New York: Simon & Schuster.

Eddy, Mary Baker. 1934. *Science and Health with Key to the Scriptures*. Boston: Trustees of Mary Baker Eddy.

Eder, Bruce. 1987. 'Keep Your Bodily Fluids to Yourself! Morton Downey Jr Slaps Gay Activist.' *Voice* (29 December):13.

Edwards, George. 1989. 'A Critique of Creationist Homophobia.' *Homosexuality and Religion*, edited by Richard Hasbany. New York: Harrington Park Press.

Ellis, Carl F., Jr. 1983. *Beyond Liberation: The Gospel in the Black American Experience*. Downers Grove, IL: InterVarsity.

Ellwood, Robert S. 1973. *Religious and Spiritual Groups in Modern America*. Englewood Cliffs, NJ: Prentice Hall.

Ellwood, Robert S. 1979. *Alternative Altars*. Chicago University Press.

Evans, Christopher. 1974. *Cults of Unreason*. New York: Dell Publishers.

Farber, Celia. 1991. 'Michael Callen: Surviving Is What I Do.' *Spin* 7 (1):18.

Feshuk, Scott. 1995. 'Accused Boasted of HIV Plot, Court Told.' *Globe and Mail* (10 May):A1.

Fiedler, Leslie. 1978. *Freaks*. New York: Simon & Schuster/Touchstone.

Field, Rick. 1986. *How the Swan Came to the Lake*. Boulder, CO: Shambala.

Fitterman, Lisa. 1991. 'A Wife's Terror: AIDS Allegations Means Hab Wives Have More to Worry About Than Ever.' *Ottawa Citizen*, Hockey Section (31 December):B6.

Fitzgerald, Frances. 1986. 'The Reporter at Large: Rajneeshpuram 11.' *The New Yorker* (29 September).

Fitzpatrick, Ray. 1984. 'Lay Concepts of Illness.' *The Experience of Illness.* London: Tavistock.

'Former Santa Suing Retailer over AIDS Complaint.'1994. *Montreal Gazette* (7 April):A6.

Fortunato, John E. 1987. *AIDS, the Spiritual Dilemma.* San Francisco: Harper & Row.

Foster, Lawrence. 1981. *Religion and Sexuality.* New York: Oxford University Press.

Glendon, Mary Ann. 1985. *The New Family and the New Property.* Toronto: Butterworth.

Goffman, Erving. 1968. *Stigma: Notes on the Management of Spoiled Identity.* London: Penguin Books.

Goldstein, Richard. 1987. 'AIDS and the Social Contract.' *Village Voice* (29 December):17.

Gorer, Geoffrey. 1965. *Death, Grief and Mourning in Contemporary Britain.* London: Cresset Press.

Grace, James. 1985. *Sexuality and Marriage in the Unification Church.* Toronto: Edwin Mellen Press.

Graham, Billy. 1987. 'AIDS, Sex and the Bible.' *Decision* (October).

Gray, Jerry. 1985. 'Africa: Birthplace of a Dreaded Disease?' *Houston Chronicle* (15 September).

Gregory, Stephen, & Bernard Leonardo. 1986. *Conquering AIDS Now! With Natural Treatment and the Non-Drug Approach.* New York: Warner Books.

Guerrero, Edward. 1990. 'AIDS as Monster in Horror Cinema.' *Journal of Popular Film & Television* 18(3) (Fall):86–92. Popular Culture Center, Bowling Green State University.

Hamilton, Joan. 1987. 'The AIDS Epidmic and Business.' *Business Week* (March).

Hasbany, Richard. 1989. *Homosexuality and Religion.* New York: Harrington Park.

Hay, Louise. 1987. *You Can Heal Your Life.* California: Hay House.

Hay, Louise. 1988. *The AIDS Book.* California: Hay House.

Heard, Gerald. 1987. 'A Future for the Isophyl and What Is Religion?' *Gay Spirit: Myth and Meaning,* edited by Mark Thompson. New York: St Martin's Press.

'Heartache in Happy Valley: AIDS Hits Mormon Utah.' 1988. *Montreal Gazette* (29 February):A5.

Henican, Elle. 1988. 'Dads Battle Cult for Children: Lawsuit Penetrating a Shroud of Secrecy at Sullivanian Institute.' *Newsday* (31 May).

Hey, Robert P. 1987. 'Spread of AIDS in U.S. Population Appears Limited.' *Christian Science Monitor* (26 October), National:4.

'High Life and Low Life.' 1992. *Vogue* (November).

Hinkley, Gordon B. 1987. 'Reverence and Morality.' *Ensign Magazine* (May).

'Homosexuality: Nature Never Produces Anything Which Is Useless.' 1988. *Rajneesh Times International* (1 March).

Hopp, Joyce W. 1986. 'AIDS: The Up-and-Coming Disease,' and 'AIDS: What Should We Do?' *Adventist Review* (September):8.

Hughes, Ted. 1992. 'The Fraying of America.' 1992. *Time* (3 February):46.

Judah, J. Stillson. 1967. *The History and Philosophy of the Metaphysical Movements in America*. Philadelphia: Westminster.

Judah, Stillson. 1974. *The Hare Krishna and the Counter Culture*. New York: John Wiley & Sons.

Kanter, Rosabeth Moss. 1972. *Commitment and Community: Communes and Utopias in Sociological Perspective*. Cambridge, MA: Harvard University Press.

Kayal, Philip M. 1989. 'Healing as Political Innovation.' Paper presented at the October Meeting of the Society for the Scientific Study of Religion in Salt Lake City.

Kern, Louis. 1981. *An Ordered Love*. Chapel Hill: University of North Carolina Press.

'Kill AIDS Victims – Muslim Cleric.' 1989. *The Nairobi Standard* (4 July):26.

King, Dennis, & Ronald Radosh. 1984. 'The LaRouche Connection.' *New Republic* (19 November):15.

Klimo, Jon. 1987. *Channeling: Investigations on Receiving Information from Paranormal Sources*. Los Angeles: Jeremy P. Tarcher.

Koop, Everett. 1986. *Surgeon General's Report on AIDS (Acquired Immune Deficiency Syndrome)*. P.O. Box 14252, Washington, DC, 20044.

Koshland, Daniel, Jr. 1987. 'Epidemics and Civil Rights.' *Science* 235(4790) (13 February):729.

Kübler-Ross, Elizabeth. 1987. *AIDS: The Ultimate Challenge*. New York: Macmillan.

Lanphear, Roger G. 1990. *Gay Spirituality*. San Diego: Unified Publications.

LaRouche, Lyndon. 1987. *The Power of Reason: 1988*. Washington, DC: Executive Intelligence Review.

'LaRouche Warns Spread Panic, Not AIDS.' (n.d.) *National Democratic Policy Committee*. Washington, DC.

Lasch, Christopher. 1978. *The Culture of Narcissism*. New York: Norton.

Lattin, Don. 1989a. 'Sex, AIDS Scandal Forces Buddhist Leader into Retreat.' *San Francisco Chronicle* (18 February):18–19.

Lattin, Don. 1989b. 'Hayrides and Healing in the Castro.' *San Francisco Chronicle* (27 February):16.

Lee, Martha F. 1995. *Earth First! Environmental Apocalypse*. New York: Syracuse University Press.

Lewin, Tamar. 1988. 'Custody Case Lifts Veil on a Psychotherapy Cult.' *New York Times* (28 May):B1.

Lewis, James R., & J. Gordon Melton, eds. 1994. *Church Universal and Triumphant in Scholarly Perspective*. Stanford, CA: Centre for Academic Publication.

Lewis, Richard R. 1990. 'AIDS: Scourge of the 20th, Healer of the 21st?' *Unification News* (November):24.

Lippe, Toinette. 1995. 'Ma Jaya from the Holy Lande of Brooklyn.' *Shambala Sun* (March).

Lippy, Edward. 1989. *Twentieth-Century Shapers of American Popular Religion*. New York: Greenwood Press.

Mada, Ma Jivan. 1990. 'The Only AIDS-free Zone in the World: The Osho International Commune.' Paper presented at the *Religion and AIDS* Symposium (1 April), McGill University, Montreal.

Mains, Geoff. 1987. 'Urban Aboriginals and the Celebration of Leather Magic.' *Gay Spirit, Myth and Meaning*, edited by Mark Thompson. New York: St Martin's Press.

Manes, Christopher. 1987. 'Miss An Thropy Responds to Alien Nation.' *Earth First!* 8(2) (22 December):17.

Mankoff, Martin. 1971. 'Societal Reaction and Career Deviance: A Critical Analysis.' *Sociological Quarterly* 12:214–18.

Markoff Asistent, Niro. 1991. 'Why I Survive AIDS.' *New Age Journal* (September/October):38.

Martin, William. 1982. 'Waiting for the End.' *The Atlantic* (June).

Mayer, Jean-Francois. 1994. 'Les Schismes de l' Église Universelle de Dieu.' *Mouvements Religieux* (July). Sarreguemines, Switzerland, 2–7.

Melton, J. Gordon. 1986. *The Encyclopedic Handbook of Cults in America*. New York: Garland.

Melton, J. Gordon. 1989. *The Churches Speak on AIDS*. Detroit: Gale Research Inc.

Melton, J. Gordon. 1995. 'Sexuality and the Maturation of the Family.' *Sex, Slander and Salvation*, edited by James R. Lewis and J. Gordon Melton. Golito, CA: University Press of America.

Melton, J. Gordon. 'Finding Enlightenment with Ramtha: The Emergence of Gnosticism in the West.' Unpublished manuscript.

Methvin, Eugene. 1986. 'Lyndon LaRouche's Raid on Democracy.' *Reader's Digest* (August):90.

Miller, James. 1993. *The Passion of Michel Foucault*. New York: Simon & Schuster.

Mitchell, Alanna. 1995. 'Tan Not Guilty of Injecting Lover.' *Globe and Mail* (24 May):A5.

Monnette, Paul. 1990. *Borrowed Time: An AIDS Memoir*. New York: Avon Books.

Monnette, Paul. (n.d.) *Last Watch of the Night: Essays Too Personal and Otherwise.'* New York: Harcourt Brace.

Moon, Reverend Sun Myung. 1987. 'Let Us Go Over the Original Boundary.' Talk given 1 April at Belvedere, CA, Translator, Bo Hi Pak.

Moore, Lawrence R. 1977. *In Search of White Crows: Spiritualism, Parapsychology and American Culture*. New York: Oxford University Press.

Moritz, William. 1987. 'Seven Glimpses of Walt Whitman.' *Gay Spirit: Myth and Meaning*, edited by Mark Thompson. New York: St Martin's Press.

Morrison, Ken. 1988. 'Sexual Healing: AIDS-Prevention Programs by Our Ministries of Health Have So Far Been Mostly Talk.' *Montreal Mirror* (15 December):5.

Myler, Kathleen. 1988. 'AIDS in the Workplace: Major Firms Combat Fears with Compassion.' *Houston Chronicle* (1 May), Section 9:1.

'Names Project Plans Display of Entire AIDS Memorial Quilt in Washington, DC.' 1995. *The Quilt News* (May).

Palmer, Susan. 1986. 'Purity and Danger in the Rajneesh Foundation.' Update (August), Aarhus, Denmark.

Palmer, Susan. 1989. 'Virus as Metaphor: Religious Responses to AIDS.' *In Gods We Trust*, edited by Tom Robbins. NJ: Transaction.

Patton, Cindy. 1986. *Sex and Germs: The Politics of AIDS*. Montreal & Buffalo: Black Rose Books.

Pearls of Wisdom. Newsletter. The Summit University Press, Box A, Livingston, MT 59047-1390.

Pearson, Michael. 1990. *Millennial Dreams and Moral Dilemmas*. New York: Cambridge University Press.

Penn, Kristin. 1989. 'Meditation and AIDS: A Return to Wholeness.' *Karuna: A Journal of Buddhist Meditation* 6(1) (Spring):13.

Perlez, Jane. 1991. 'Ugandan Wife Confronts a Custom to Avoid AIDS.' *New York Times* (2 March):2.

Philips, Abn Ameenah Bilal. 1988. *The Ansaar Cult in America*. Riyadh, Saudi Arabia: Tawheed.

Phinney, Allison W., Jr. 1988. 'Something Must be Done, Something We Can Do." *Christian Science Sentinel* 90(15) (11 April):25.

'Plague to AIDS: Lessons from Our Past.' 1990. (Review of an exhibit at the Museum of the History of Medicine.) *Ontario Medicine* (21 May):33.

Platt, John. 1987. 'The Future of AIDS.' 1987. *Futurist* (November/December):10–17. World Future Society, Bethesda, MD.

Poleman, Dick. 1986. 'Way Bandy: The Famous Makeup Artist Keeps His Life Public but Wants His Death Private.' *US Magazine* 3(37) (17 November):48.

'Professor Sees AIDS as Punishing Homosexuals.' 1992. *Ottawa Citizen*
   (3 May):A9.

Prophet, Elizabeth Clare. 1986. *St Germain on Prophecy*. Livingston, MT: Summit
   University Press.

Prophet, Mark L. 1981. *The Soulless One: Cloning a Counterfeit Creation*.
   Livingston, MT: Summit University Press.

Rael. 1989. *The Message Given to Me by Extraterrestrials*. Tokyo: Raelian
   Foundation.

Rajneesh, Bhagwan Shree. 1985. 'Follow AIDS Prevention Measures or Suffer.'
   The Rajneesh Times AIDS Watch. (18 October).

Rajneesh, Bhagwan Shree. 1988. 'Homosexuality Is Useless.' *Rajneesh Times*.
   Discourse 6 (20 January).

Rajneesh, Bhagwan Shree. 1988. 'Homosexuality.' *Rajneesh Times* 5(6)
   (1 March):10.

Ramtha. 1987. *Intensive Change: The Days Yet to Come*. Eastsound, WA:
   Sovereignty, Inc.

River Fund. Newsletter. 11155 Roseland Road, Unit 16. Sebastian, FL.

Robbins, Tom. 1988. *Cults, Converts and Charisma*. Beverly Hills, CA: Sage.

'Rock Hudson.' 1988. *People* (Fall):65–6.

Rogers, Deborah. 1988. 'AIDS Spreads to the Soaps, Sort Of.' *New York Times*
   (28 August 1988): Section H.

Saharan, Pawan K. (n.d.) 'AIDS: A Shastric Perspective.' *Bhaktivedanta Institute
   Bulletin* 9(4/5).

Satuloff, Bob. 1991. 'Taking Poison: An Interview with Filmmaker Todd
   Haynes.' *Rialto: Montreal's Repertory Cinema*. 2(3) (31 May):11.

Schecter, Stephen. 1990. *The AIDS Notebooks*. Albany: State University of New
   York.

Schioler, Karen Capen. 1988. 'AIDS: Sexual Expression, Social Violence.'
   Unpublished manuscript.

Schmidt, Eric. 'Church and State Clash Over AIDS Education – Plymouth
   Brethren.' *New York Times* (8 January 1990).

Schoofs, Mark. 1994. 'Love Stories in the Age of AIDS.' *Village Voice* 39(33)
   (16 August):23.

Schwartz, Gary. 1970. *Sect Ideologies and Social Status*. Chicago: University of
   Chicago Press.

Schwartz, Paul. 1989. 'Solitude, Not Exile.' Unpublished manuscript.

Scrambler, Graham. 1991. 'Stigmatizing Illness.' *The New Modern Sociology
   Readings*, edited by Peter Worseley. London: Penguin Books.

Sesser, Stan. 1994. 'Hidden Death: Why Are Some Japanese Leaving Their

Nation to Die Abroad? Many People with AIDS Feel They Have No Other Choice.' *The New Yorker* (14 November):62.

Shapiro, Walter, & Gerald C. Lumenow. 1986. 'Lyndon RaRouche; Beyond the Fringe. *Newsweek* (7 April):38.

Shepherd, Harvey. 1987. 'Condom Advertising Isn't the Antidote to AIDS, Says Bishop.' *Montreal Gazette* (14 March):J5.

Sherrill, Martha. 'A Course in Marianne.' *Mirabella* (April 1994):132.

Shilts, Randy. 1987. 'A Devastating Look at the Politics of AIDS.' (Review of *And the Band Played On: Politics, People and the AIDS Epidemic.*) *Chicago Tribune* (18 October).

'Shock Treatment – Robert Mapplethorpe.' 1990. *Montreal Mirror* (22 March).

Smelgis, Martha. 1987. 'The Big Chill: How Heterosexuals Are Coping with AIDS.' *Time* (16 February).

Sontag, Susan. 1978. *Illness as Metaphor.* New York: Vintage Books.

Sontag, Susan. 1989. *AIDS and Its Metaphors.* New York: Anchor.

'Soviets Are Running the AIDS Coverup!' 1985. *Executive Intelligence Review.* (18 October).Washington, DC: LaRouchians.

Stone, Donald. 1976. 'The Human Potential Movement.' *The New Religious Consciousness,* edited by Charles Glock and Robert Bellah. Berkeley: University of California Press.

Stone, Lawrence. 1977. *Family, Sex, and Marriage in England, 1500–1800.* New York: Harper & Row.

Stoner, J.B. (n.d.) 'Letter to Pastor Richard G. Butler.' *Aryan Nations: Calling Our Nation,* No. 52.

'Surviving Is What I Do: Doctors Puzzle Over Why Some AIDS Sufferers Can Hang on to Life.' 1988. *Time* (2 May):58.

'Tale of Revenge Stirs AIDS Furor: Woman Claims She's Trying to Infect Men, Prompting a Surge of Concern.' 1991. *New York Times* (18 October): Nation A16.

Thompson, Mark. 1987. *Gay Spirit: Myth and Meaning.* New York: St Martin's Press.

Trungpa, Chogyam. 1974. *Born in Tibet.* Boulder, CO: Shambala.

'UFO Aliens Are Spreading AIDS: They're Using the Disease to Take Over the Planet!' 1988. *Examiner* (5 July):7.

Urbanoski, Sheila. 1990. 'Shock Treatment: Robert Mapplethorpe Jolted an Artistic World Where Shock Value Is Usually Synonymous with Price Tags.' *Montreal Mirror* (22 March):11.

'U.S. Buddhist Sect's Head Passes AIDS to Students.' 1989. *Hinduism Today* (April):3.

Vespa, Mary. 1988. 'The Quiet Victories of Ryan White.' *People* (30 May):21.

Wallis, Roy. 1975. *Sectarianism*. New York: Halstead.

Wallis, Roy. 1977. *The Road to Total Freedom*. New York: Columbia University Press.

Wallis, Roy. 1979. *Salvation and Protest*. London: Francis Pinter.

Wallis, Roy. 1984. *The Elementary Forms of the New Religious Life*. London: Routledge and Kegan Paul.

Watanabe, Teresa. 1988. 'Heartache in Happy Valley: AIDS Hits Mormon Utah.' *Montreal Gazette* (29 February):A5.

Weigert, Andrew J. 1988. 'Christian Eschatology in Nuclear Context.' *Journal for the Scientific Study of Religion* 27(2).

Wessinger, Catherine, ed. 1993. *Women's Leadership in Marginal Religions: Explorations Outside the Mainstream*. Urbana & Chicago: University of Illinois Press.

Westley, Frances. 1979. 'Purity, Danger and Facelessness.' *Studies in Religion/ Sciences Religeuses*.

Westley, Frances. 1983. *The Complex Forms of Religious Life*. Chico, CA: Scholars Press.

White, A.V. 1965. *A History of the Warfare of Science with Theology*. New York: Free Press.

White, T. 1967. *A People for His Name*. New York: Vantage Press.

Whitman, David. 1991. 'Working Magic in the Inner City.' *U.S. News and World Report* (18 November):82.

Wuthnow, Robert. 1989. *The Restructuring of American Religion*. Princeton, NJ: Princeton University Press.

Yadharani, Devi Dasi. 1990. 'AIDS: Incurable Disease with an International Passport.' Paper presented at *Religion and AIDS* Symposium (1 April), McGill University, Montreal.

Zeigler, Philip. 1971. *The Black Death*. New York: Harper & Row, Publishers.

Index